When Ministry Meets Medicine

A Modern Motivational Journal for Holistic Wellness

Andrea Green Willis, M.D., MPH, FAAP, with Pastor Antoyne Green

They Speak Publishing

Dallas, Texas

When Ministry Meets Medicine
A Modern Motivational Journal for Holistic Wellness

Published by They Speak Publishing, Dallas, Texas
www.theyspeakpublishing.com

Headshots by Sergio Plecas and Portrait Innovations, respectively.

Printed in the United States of America
978-0-578-59912-0

Dedication

This journal is dedicated to our family. We come from people who were not shy about expressing their perspectives. Even though our grandparents, Willie and Rosie French and Friend and Fannie Green, are no longer with us, the memories of who they were and what they stood for still motivate us.

To our parents, Deloris and George Green (who are also not shy), thank you for nurturing our talents and encouraging us to use our voices. This book is just one example of that. We cannot thank you enough.

Andrea: I also want to dedicate this journal to my son, Cam. I thank God for the blessing you are. You motivate me in so many ways. I cannot wait to see the great things you will do in this world. Love you much.

Antoyne: Of course, I have to take the time to thank "My Crew" for your support of my ministry for all of these years. It's one thing to be called by God to do something. It's another thing to be blessed by Him with connections to people who love and support you and your vision. So to Felicia, Jasmynn, Kaleb, and Emani, thanks so much. This journal is dedicated to each of you. Love ya'll!

Contents

Foreword

I believe we are born to solve a problem in the earth. It is that belief that has me overjoyed at this book. Serving as a pastor for over 25 years and being married to a physician, I know the challenges of merging the two disciplines. For years, the faith community has downplayed and even demonized the role of medicine where healing is concerned. There are statements spoken across pulpits that declare "the doctor is a liar, believe God." Conversely, there are shared sentiments from the medical profession that have minimized the role of faith and spirituality in the lives of people in relationship to their health care. This problem in the earth has been appropriately addressed by what I consider two very capable professionals. This journal is life changing and will help the medical and faith community find common ground when addressing issues of health and wellness.

Medicine and faith can work together. Medicine provides factual information regarding diagnosis and gives prognosis based on the data available to them. In order for faith to function, it must begin where facts end. The two are not mutually exclusive from each other. The risk we run when we do not yield to the wisdom of those assigned to us in the medical profession is creating a culture where people refuse necessary treatment that could save their lives. We create a culture where people refuse to take their medicine, believing God will just heal them. I more than many believe God is a healer, yet I also understand what the scriptures says in James 2:17, "Faith without works is dead." Faith requires a corresponding action that positions us as believers to work with God rather than against Him.

It's only until we accept that medical professionals, just like clergy, can be used by God, that we will begin to see an effective merger of the two fields. God gives physicians the wisdom to do what they do and you the faith to trust His word for the results. This journal is written to help us all reconcile the tension between our faith and the facts medicine presents to us daily. If you take your time, process each page and point, it will help you live a life of balance where these two areas are concerned. This journal is an answer to many prayers. I know it will bless you.

Bishop Joseph Warren Walker, III
Senior Pastor at Mount Zion Baptist Church, Nashville, TN
Presiding Bishop of the Full Gospel Baptist Church Fellowship

Introduction

I believe the church, specifically some of the behaviors perpetuated in the church, is killing the congregants. Okay, maybe that is severe. Put another way, is the church truly promoting health? Before you throw this book away and start thinking harshly of me, I believe the church is powerful. However, I think it has used its power selectively. For example, many times I have heard, "We are praying together and coming against cancer." I am not opposed to this. However, why aren't we coming against obesity? And what about heart disease? It kills more people than cancer and disproportionately affects people of color. Why aren't coming against heart disease? Is it because we're not willing to change our behaviors, some of which are practiced within the church? Some of the best fried-food dinners are held at church! Yes, it tastes good, but we know that it is not good for us.

Why aren't we coming against depression and other mental illnesses? Why do so many people suffer daily believing that they have to pray mental illness away? Why aren't people hearing from the pulpit that it is okay to get help? Why aren't people seeing healthy preachers behind the podiums? We can literally see that many preachers are not practicing what they preach. Doesn't 3 John: 2 (KJV) say, "Beloved, I wish above all things that thou mayest prosper and be in health, even as thy soul prospereth"?

I remember studying for Step 3 of my boards years ago. A question asked, "What is it called when a diabetic knowingly and consistently indulges in behaviors that raise his/her blood sugar?" The answer surprised me. It said the person is committing chronic suicide. I am not telling you that you have to accept that answer. What I am telling you is that I can't forget that answer. But if we suppose for a second that the answer is correct, is the church an accomplice? Is the church loving us to death?

I am a Christian. My faith is in God. He has blessed me and has shown me favor. I am also a doctor. My goal of being provocative in my opening statement is actually my way of trying to give back. I want to jolt you into action! It is meant to stir discussion in the church that will result in the church meaningfully wielding its power to make its congregants whole in body, mind, and spirit.

I am co-writing this book with my brother who is a pastor. I believe in his anointing. I also believe that I am called to ministry as well, although not in the same way he is—hence, the title of the book. I have had fights within myself when it has seemed at times that medicine and ministry collide. I have found peace and realize that medicine is my ministry. However, the heated arguments between my brother and I can go to the next level and can be epic at times.

In the past, he has asked me for a medical prognosis regarding a congregant or relative. If my response was that the diagnosis was terminal, he would wonder, "Where was your faith?"

My response would be, "You asked me the medical prognosis. I gave you that." In no way does that speak to my faith or rather a lack of faith. I would tell him, "At least I know what I'm praying for." I would sarcastically think, "You do your job, preacher, and let me do mine."

We recognize that we both want the same thing. That's why we are writing this book. We believe medicine and ministry, when in sync, can positively change lives. I believe that God does heal through medicine. However, there are times that medicine has done all that it can do. At those times, God either heals miraculously or He heals on the other side.

This book is meant to let you into our arguments. We want to be real and let you hear varied perspectives. More importantly, we want you to see the resolution of those arguments. We want the same outcome. Our approaches are different. That just means there is an opportunity to open our minds to hear a different side. We grow that way.

We have organized this publication as a journal to keep you engaged throughout the year. It takes weeks to sustain behavior change. Through this format, we hope we can support your journey. At the beginning of each month, we will give you some narrative for thought. You will hear my perspective, labeled *medicine*, and you will hear my brother's perspective, labeled *ministry*. We cannot tell you what's right. Hopefully, we can help you find out what's right for you.

How This Journal Works

We have supplied you with enough pages to journal every day. The first page of each month's journal pages will prompt you to set goals for the month. It's also a good way to track progress for year-long goals. We've included daily thoughts and vignettes to keep you motivated. The daily passages are written by me and some are written by my brother. Others are a compilation of both of our thoughts. You'll probably be able to guess which of us wrote some of them. Other times, we think you would be totally surprised by who wrote it. The point is to show that we're all in this together. We hope to guide you through a productive, faith-filled, and healthy year. Even if you didn't get this journal in time to start off in January, you can jump right in whenever you get it. Starting in January will increase your chances of starting new habits early on and maintaining them as you approach the end of the year. The most important thing is that you stay with it. Thank you for taking this journey with us.

Vision Statement

What will you accomplish this year? Go ahead and put it out there and claim it! What is your vision statement for the year ahead? What are you going to make happen? How will you be well in body, mind, and spirit to optimize your chances for achieving success? Mental, physical, and spiritual health not only augment each other but they are powerful when aligned. Commit to unleashing that power!

Are you not sure how to craft a vision statement? A vision statement documents current and future objectives. It aligns with your philosophy. It sets your strategy. It stretches you and inspires you. Here are some popular vision statements crafted by companies with which we are familiar:

Nike: "Bring inspiration and innovation to every athlete* in the world. (*If you have a body, you are an athlete.)"

Southwest Airlines: "To become the world's most loved, most flown, and most profitable airline."

Do these organizations live up to their vision statements? They put them out there to hold themselves accountable and for us to hold them accountable as well. Now it's your turn.

My vision statement for this year:

_____

_____

_____

_____

_____

_____

_____

January

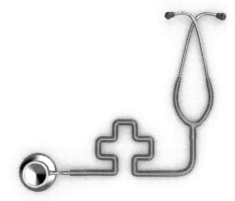

January
Revelation Versus Resolution

Medicine

January is the month in which we start with new resolutions. This year, I'm going to lose weight. This year, I'm going to read my Bible more. This year, I'm going to let go of toxic relationships.

We say that it's a new beginning, but in the crevices of our minds, I believe there are nagging questions. How did I get here? Is it really about grasping a new beginning or letting go of old habits and demons? I believe we do have to face our pasts so that we don't repeat them. More important is that we don't get bogged down on how we got where we are. Instead, we should use that experience as a stepping stone to get out of our current situation. What I know for sure is that you can't do the same thing and think there will be a different result.

I know of people who are diabetics who believe by faith they will come off of their medications. They believe this while they eat sweet potato pie. I don't have to tell you what's wrong with that picture. There are diagnoses such as diabetes, obesity, and countless other diseases that can be improved by eating better and being physically active. However, often people choose not to be intentional about a healthier lifestyle. For conditions influenced by lifestyle, I do not believe that faith alone will reverse the illness. Changing a lifestyle is not at all easy. Frederick Douglass said, "If there is no struggle, there is no progress." This is a place where we can exercise faith both figuratively and literally. Faith without works is dead. Isn't that right, preacher?

Ministry

It is true that faith without works is dead. However, I also believe that works without faith are most often fruitless. Faith is the foundation—the infrastructure—on which believers build their lives. This is true in every facet of life imaginable: spiritually, mentally, emotionally, physically, financially, professionally, relationally, and otherwise.

Faith has so many levels. By faith, we believe that God exists and is Creator and Ruler of all things. Our saving faith says we believe God sent His son Jesus as our Savior to die, to be buried, and to be resurrected to save us from the penalty of sin and power of sin. Then, there is a sustaining faith that believes God can and will do what we need Him to do, desire Him to do, and ask Him to do.

All three levels of faith are crucial in making life decisions about health—among other things. The struggles people have taking control of each facet of their lives are real. I agree that we should reflect on our past without returning and residing there. However, it's easier said than done. For many people, the past has, in essence, arrested their bodies, minds, emotions, spirits, and determination. It takes faith to even begin the process of seeing oneself better than what one's present state suggests.

I also agree that a diabetic eating sweet potato pie is counterproductive. However, for some, it's the pie, the cake, the huge meals, the alcohol, or countless other foods and drinks where, unfortunately, they've found their comfort and dependence. It will take every aspect of faith just to refocus and regroup. It will take one's faith to believe that one can make the transition to good health and healthy habits. It will take faith (and time) for that person to fully rely on God to sustain him or her in the process.

It's easy for doctors or family to say, "You need to…" However, I contend that there must be great consideration, beyond science *and* beyond religious rhetoric, given to a person who is struggling with his or her health or otherwise. That person must reach deep in faith to align the "you need to" with "God, I need you to." It's on God upon whom we must fully rely. With Him, all things really are possible.

January

This is your new start! What are your goals for January?

1.

2.

3.

January 1st

Thought of the Day

Don't let "Happy New Year" just be a saying. Let it be your reality. Let's start the year off right. As you navigate the journey to a healthier life, don't compare yourself to others. You are your own best measuring stick for your success. One size does not fit all. The question that you should really answer along with your primary care provider is, "What should be my goals to optimize my health?" Knowing your destination helps you to set your path. Invoking your faith will help push you along that path.

My prayer for today is:

_____

_____

_____

What I will do today to be active in starting this year off right:

_____

_____

_____

_____

My thoughts for today:

_____

_____

_____

_____

_____

January 2ⁿᵈ

Thought of the Day

It's never too late! Check out the story of Ernestine Shepherd. She's a body builder in her 80's. She began working out in her 50's. She looks remarkable. Her work ethic is extremely disciplined. If you want a better life, you've got to improve your living! There's a no better time to get started than today—no matter your age.

My prayer for today is:

_____

_____

_____

What I will do today to be active in starting this year off right:

_____

_____

_____

_____

My thoughts for today:

_____

_____

_____

_____

January 3rd

Thought of the Day

I was doing a half marathon in Tucson. There was a boy with cerebral palsy running with his dad. I encountered them at around mile 8. As he ran by my side, he said, "You rock." It was so unexpected, but it encouraged me greatly. I told him that he was the one who rocked. I wanted to see him finish well. I started to leave he and his dad when he began to tire. I still had great energy, and I knew he wouldn't want anyone to slow down for him. At mile 10, I started to tire and the boy and his dad started to catch up. My prayer at that point was that God grant him favor to give him a second wind to finish the race. From there on, I ran slightly behind them. It did my heart good to see him cross that line and the excitement that ensued. In my mind, I was watching scripture unfold. "But they that wait upon the Lord shall renew their strength; they shall mount up with wings like eagles; they shall run and not be weary, and they shall walk, and not faint" (Isaiah 40:31, KJV). Just bearing witness to someone else who makes it through the struggle is a win for everyone in the race. All of your motivation doesn't come before the race. Sometimes it comes in the race.

My prayer for today is:

_____

_____

_____

What I will do today to be active in starting this year off right:

_____

_____

_____

_____

My thoughts for today:

_____

_____

_____

_____

_____

January 4th

Thought of the Day

Everybody is talking about how their NEXT is going to be so great. That's cool. But never forget that RIGHT NOW is the only guaranteed time we have. Therefore, NOW is the season to be sure of yourself and make every second count. The discipline, decisions, determination, discernment, and focus of NOW are the only things that really matter.

My prayer for today is:

_____

_____

_____

What I will do today to be active in starting this year off right:

_____

_____

_____

_____

My thoughts for today:

_____

_____

_____

_____

January 5th

Thought of the Day

Picture yourself when you reach your goal. During my first 5K, I met a lady who said she got into running as she was going through a nasty divorce. She said that when she started she would walk and cry. Then she began to walk and pray. Soon after, she would jog and pray. After she became more fit, she started to lift weights, and she would pray then too. She went on to win fitness competitions. When she started off, her goal was just to feel better emotionally. She ended up being whole in body, mind, and spirit. Your goal doesn't have to be singular in focus but it should include being better than where you started.

My prayer for today is:

_____

_____

_____

What I will do today to be active in starting this year off right:

_____

_____

_____

_____

My thoughts for today:

_____

_____

_____

_____

_____

January 6th

Thought of the Day

When you expect great things, your mind and your heart won't let you settle for just anything! Friend, keep your focus on the favor from God that's on its way to your life! He has blessed you with another year. There is no reason to believe that it will be anything less than a great one. When we say, "Get active," that applies to a lot of things. Get physically active, but get active in your prayer life, too. Get active in making yourself a priority. If you take one step, He'll take two. Start this year off the way you want to finish it—strong.

My prayer for today is:

_____

_____

_____

What I will do today to be active in starting this year off right:

_____

_____

_____

_____

My thoughts for today:

_____

_____

_____

_____

_____

January 7th

Thought of the Day

Sometimes we are so determined to come out of the gate swinging that we start off too fast and then burn out. We want to look great instantly after we start exercising so we exercise in the morning and in the evening and only drink veggie juice in between. After a week, we're ready to throw in the towel because it was too much too soon. We take on a new job, and we work until 10 pm every night and on the weekends to show our worth. It's not too long before we're crying about work-life balance. Don't start off sprinting if the goal is to run a marathon. Keep your eyes on the prize, but set a pace that you can sustain.

My prayer for today is:

_____

_____

_____

What I will do today to be active in starting this year off right:

_____

_____

_____

_____

My thoughts for today:

_____

_____

_____

_____

January 8th

Thought of the Day

God doesn't always need us to see where He's leading us. Instead, He just wants us to remember that He's the one doing the leading. The words of the old church deacon are true, "Lord, if you lead us, we'll be led right. And if you guide, we shall not go astray." Friend, follow and lift the One who leads you each day.

My prayer for today is:

_____

_____

_____

What I will do today to be active in starting this year off right:

_____

_____

_____

My thoughts for today:

_____

_____

_____

_____

January 9th

Thought of the Day

The best inventions are born from the individuals trying to solve a problem. They come out of necessity. The best result doesn't come from people contemplating how much money they can make. It comes from designing something that can help them and others overcome a challenge. As you are embarking on a healthier you, what issues are you trying to address? That's what will keep you on course. It may not be enough to want to look good for an event. That motivation will come and go. If you are trying to get healthy so that you can potentially stop taking medications or to avoid having to start medications, that motivation will help you to invent the new you.

My prayer for today is:

_____

_____

_____

What I will do today to be active in starting this year off right:

_____

_____

_____

_____

My thoughts for today:

_____

_____

_____

_____

January 10th

Thought of the Day

There's even an app for that! There are actually many exercise apps to give people variety in their exercise routines. They even demonstrate how to do the exercises. People often fail in establishing exercise routines because they get bored. You have the ability to change it up even if you don't use an app. Walk or run today. Join a group class tomorrow. Lift weights the next day. The only thing that has to be routine is your commitment to changing your life. Pray and press your way through. You can do it!

My prayer for today is:

_____

_____

_____

What I will do today to be active in starting this year off right:

_____

_____

_____

_____

My thoughts for today:

_____

_____

_____

_____

_____

January 11ᵗʰ

Thought of the Day

Never let other people's demands and expectations on your life destroy your concentration, confidence, character, and consistency. Know that you will never be able to control the thoughts or opinions of others. Therefore, do your best. Give your all. Please God. Please yourself. And then let the chips fall where they may. You can only do what you can do. Make it a MARVELOUS day!

My prayer for today is:

_____

_____

_____

What I will do today to be active in starting this year off right:

_____

_____

_____

_____

My thoughts for today:

_____

_____

_____

_____

_____

January 12th

Thought of the Day

Your perspective directly affects your patience, your progression, and your productivity. The best view comes from a mind, heart, and eyes that are forward focused by faith. Keep looking ahead on this BLESSED day.

My prayer for today is:

_____

_____

_____

What I will do today to be active in starting this year off right:

_____

_____

_____

_____

My thoughts for today:

_____

_____

_____

_____

_____

January 13th

Thought of the Day

If the very thought of getting started on this wellness journey is making you question yourself and wonder if you can do it, let your warm-up include a prayer. When you truly trust God, you have a nine-word, three-sentence prayer: "God, I can't. But you can. Do it, Lord!" PRAY and PREVAIL on this wonderful day.

My prayer for today is:

_____

_____

_____

What I will do today to be active in starting this year off right:

_____

_____

_____

_____

My thoughts for today:

_____

_____

_____

_____

_____

January 14th

Thought of the Day

Understand that some people will never embrace your vision of who you are becoming, where you're going, and the successes awaiting you in the future because they're too fixated on your past. That's cool. You keep it moving. Don't let their obsession with your yesterday be a deterrent to your tomorrow!

My prayer for today is:

_____

_____

_____

What I will do today to be active in starting this year off right:

_____

_____

_____

_____

My thoughts for today:

_____

_____

_____

_____

_____

January 15th

Thought of the Day

If you're among those who believe that the best of your life is yet to come, be sure not to miss golden "God opportunities" in your future by continually fretting and being in self-pity about what did or didn't happen in your past. In some seasons, you'll just learn to rise up, let some things be, and focus on what's yet to come! Make it a marvelous year!

My prayer for today is:

_____

_____

_____

What I will do today to be active in starting this year off right:

_____

_____

_____

_____

My thoughts for today:

_____

_____

_____

_____

_____

January 16th

Thought of the Day

Thanks so much for another day, another year. I ask You today, dear God, to bless my friends and family. I ask you to please help my loved ones to challenge their challenges by faith and to defeat their demons by your power. All the while, Holy Father, elevate them above their enemies and every plot and plan their enemies have against their lives. And God, I ask that You bless me also as I seek to glorify You by the life I live this year. I ask these things in the name of Jesus. Amen.

My prayer for today is:

_____

_____

_____

What I will do today to be active in starting this year off right:

_____

_____

_____

_____

My thoughts for today:

_____

_____

_____

_____

_____

January 17th

Thought of the Day

One of the barriers to exercise is that it can feel like a boring routine. It is work. There is no reason that work can't be fun though. Any time your work aligns with your mission, it becomes a means to an end. The right mindset is instrumental in exercise. It fuels the will to keep going. What if you use your exercise time as prayer or meditation time? It makes a difference! I do it often. It gives you power to keep going. Exercise your faith while you exercise your body.

My prayer for today is:

_____

_____

_____

What I will do today to be active in starting this year off right:

_____

_____

_____

My thoughts for today:

_____

_____

_____

_____

_____

January 18th

Thought of the Day

Don't give up even if you slip up. Sometimes we can be doing great on our lifestyle change. We've been eating right and we've been exercising. Then we may go on a trip, or some circumstance throws us off a few days. Sometimes we'll be so disappointed that we want to lapse back to our old ways. Life happens! We would never tell people battling addictions that if they fall off the wagon, stay off the wagon. As the song *We Fall Down* says, "We fall down but we get up." Get up and keep going!

My prayer for today is:

_____

_____

_____

What I will do today to be active in starting this year off right:

_____

_____

_____

_____

My thoughts for today:

_____

_____

_____

_____

_____

January 19th

Thought of the Day

As a kid, I hated Brussels sprouts, as well as soybeans. I didn't eat them for many years because the 8-year-old me didn't like them. Wouldn't you know they are now on the menus of restaurants everywhere? Well, the soybeans go by the fancier name of edamame, but they're still soybeans. And guess what? I really like them! Be open to trying new things that could be good for you. Palates change! You don't have to be afraid of change when you have your foundation in God who doesn't change. He has you covered. Now, the day awaits. Get to it!

My prayer for today is:

_____

_____

_____

What I will do today to be active in starting this year off right:

_____

_____

_____

_____

My thoughts for today:

_____

_____

_____

_____

_____

January 20th

Thought of the Day

We stretch ourselves too thin so many times. We are double and triple booked. We take part in things in which we really have no interest. Our hearts are in the right places, but we can run ourselves ragged and not look out for own well-being. "No" is an answer. True friends and family, while they may not like it, can respect it. No is a little word with powerful meaning. Learn how to add it to your vocabulary if it's not already there.

My prayer for today is:

_____

_____

_____

What I will do today to be active in starting this year off right:

_____

_____

_____

_____

My thoughts for today:

_____

_____

_____

_____

_____

January 21st

Thought of the Day

Dr. Martin Luther King, Jr. summarized the intent of this book well in this quote: "Science investigates; religion interprets. Science gives knowledge, which is power; religion gives man wisdom, which is control. Science deals mainly with facts; religion deals mainly with values. The two are not rivals." Be open to letting them peacefully coexist in your life. Not only let them coexist, let them together make your life better.

My prayer for today is:

_____

_____

_____

What I will do today to be active in starting this year off right:

_____

_____

_____

_____

My thoughts for today:

_____

_____

_____

_____

_____

January 22nd

Thought of the Day

On a wall in my workout room, I have a saying on a wall that is attributed to Lance Armstrong: "Pain is temporary. Quitting lasts forever." It's motivation for me to keep going. There are many days that I don't want to exercise, but I know if I stop for a week, I may stop for 2 weeks, which could turn into 2 months or 2 years. Things start to creep up on us with age—like slower metabolism. That's why I keep running. Just because those types of issues are creeping toward me, I don't have to slow down to let them catch me. Who's running with me?

My prayer for today is:

_____

_____

_____

What I will do today to be active in starting this year off right:

_____

_____

_____

_____

My thoughts for today:

_____

_____

_____

_____

_____

January 23rd

Thought of the Day

Have you been to a professional football game? They often call the fans the "twelfth man." All of the men on the field have a role but the role of the fans is also important. That support is so imperative that they are an honorary part of the team. They contribute to the victory. Who's on your team? Before you start a healthy lifestyle, consult your doctor. If you are afraid to go to your doctor, you may need to choose a different one. Choose the one who makes you feel that helping you along your health journey is his or her privilege. You deserve the best!

My prayer for today is:

_____

_____

_____

What I will do today to be active in starting this year off right:

_____

_____

_____

_____

My thoughts for today:

_____

_____

_____

_____

_____

January 24th

Thought of the Day

Say a prayer and set a goal! Both short-term and long-term goals are important. For example, if your long-term goal is running a 5K, but you haven't been exercising, your first goal may just be buying the proper running shoes. The second goal may be walking a half mile. The next goal may be increasing that to a full mile the following week. You gradually increase until you get to that magical number of 3.1 miles. Celebrate meeting each of the short-term goals along the way. Each of those count as victories, too!

My prayer for today is:

_____

_____

_____

What I will do today to be active in starting this year off right:

_____

_____

_____

_____

My thoughts for today:

_____

_____

_____

_____

January 25th

Thought of the Day

You are human! You can and should have a celebratory cupcake from time to time. Just make sure that it doesn't throw off your ultimate goal. Think of how to fit that into your plan. For example, I love pasta, but I know I can't have it every day. If I am going to do a long run on a Saturday, I will eat a moderate portion of pasta on Friday night. I will only eat it if I can assure myself that I will make that long run the next day. I look forward to it, and it's also part of the plan. If I hit a major milestone, I'll treat myself. You'll lose your battle with fitness if you take away everything you enjoy. It takes discipline but not deprivation. Enjoy your journey!

My prayer for today is:

_____

_____

_____

What I will do today to be active in starting this year off right:

_____

_____

_____

_____

My thoughts for today:

_____

_____

_____

_____

_____

January 26th

Thought of the Day

I'm thoroughly convinced that if many of us were as open to God as we are open to everyone on social media, many of our struggles would cease! My advice is for you to give God full access to your life so He can work on you, in you, through you, and for you. During that time, it's best that the public not be privy to what really should be held in private. You need the Father's rescue and restoration; not the folks' referendum on what's going on in your life, what you should do, and how it's going to turn out. Jesus is on the main line, not on social media.

My prayer for today is:

_____

_____

_____

What I will do today to be active in starting this year off right:

_____

_____

_____

_____

My thoughts for today:

_____

_____

_____

_____

_____

January 27th

Thought of the Day

One thing is for sure, sulking and sighing ARE NOT forward steps to surviving and succeeding. So it happened. So it turned out entirely different than expected. So it is what it is. So it really hurts. No, you're not to act as if nothing bothers you. But we must learn to have our moments, then get mentally strong in order to develop the desire, the determination, and the doubt-free spirit that will allow us to conquer every challenge. Make it a determined day!

My prayer for today is:

_____

_____

_____

What I will do today to be active in starting this year off right:

_____

_____

_____

My thoughts for today:

_____

_____

_____

_____

January 28th

Thought of the Day

I think music from the past was more impactful than a lot of the music today. Music in the past often served as the backdrop to important movements. It could motivate people to take action for positive change. When Marvin Gaye sang, "What's going on?" it promoted awareness. It seems to me old-school music was created to make us feel something and to be awake in our environment. By contrast, it seems some of today's music is created just to talk about sex and money. That's why you have to march to the beat of your own drum. Your beat should keep time with your values. You've got to know for yourself what's going on. Don't become a passive listener in a world that needs active participants. Stay woke!

My prayer for today is:

_____

_____

_____

What I will do today to be active in starting this year off right:

_____

_____

_____

My thoughts for today:

_____

_____

_____

_____

January 29th

Thought of the Day

Have you ever seen anybody ridicule somebody overweight in the gym or walking in a 5K? Your attitude should never be anything other than to help cheer others on their way. And if you are the one who is insecure in those settings, don't let a few shallow people deter you from achieving your goal. Don't let others deflect their insecurities on you. Love yourself and who you are becoming. What I love about working out is that I use that time to let God shape me while I'm getting in shape. I let Jesus work it out while I'm working out.

My prayer for today is:

_____

_____

_____

What I will do today to be active in starting this year off right:

_____

_____

_____

My thoughts for today:

_____

_____

_____

_____

January 30th

Thought of the Day

If you want to change your health for the better, you have to change your lifestyle for forever. It's about your mindset. Don't diet—eat healthy. Will you be perfect all the time? Of course not! But you can commit to eating healthier most of the time. If just the thought of exercise makes you tired, don't think of doing hard-core exercise in a gym but commit to becoming physically active. Don't set yourself up for failure with mental gymnastics! Babies crawl before they walk (most of them anyway). However, when they start to walk, we have to clear everything off of the tables because nothing can stop them from exploring their new world. They may fall, but they never look back. It's the same for you on your lifestyle journey. Start crawling. You won't automatically be your best, but you can be better!

My prayer for today is:

_____

_____

_____

What I will do today to be active in starting this year off right:

_____

_____

_____

_____

My thoughts for today:

_____

_____

_____

_____

_____

January 31st

Thought of the Day

Nine words that should encourage you to pursue your dreams and never give up—there is no limit if God is in it! Don't settle for mediocrity when you have and serve the Master who can blow your mind! Think big!

My prayer for today is:

_____

_____

_____

What I will do today to be active in starting this year off right:

_____

_____

_____

_____

My thoughts for today:

_____

_____

_____

_____

_____

February

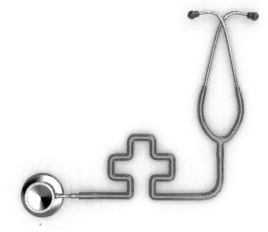

February
The Heart of the Matter

Medicine

When we think of February, we often think of Valentine's Day. Some look forward to receiving candy and flowers. Some feel sadness and spend the day trying to ignore the tokens of affection that others are receiving around them. Ironically, February is also American Heart Month, which promotes awareness of heart disease. We *Go Red for Women*. We are reminded of the statistics that heart disease is the leading cause of death for both men and women with death rates higher in people of color. We are familiar with the risk factors—overweight and obesity, diabetes, physical inactivity, and excessive alcohol use. Have we become numb to those facts? Or don't we love ourselves enough to confront the facts? That's really the heart of the matter.

There is so much in the world we can't control. Sometimes it feels like self-love even falls in that category. We can't stop the narratives or images from the media that often make us stare into the mirror and consciously or unconsciously wonder where we measure up. At those times, we have to remember to see ourselves the way God sees us. We are His children and each one of us is good enough. That doesn't stop us from striving to be our best selves. Instead, we should find strength in knowing that our Father loves us and we are worthy of being loved. That should be the basis of our loving ourselves. I love that God loves us just the way He's made us. I think that helps many of us love ourselves. How we express ourselves with our hair is just one example of us loving ourselves.

I love the natural hair movement and that it's becoming more widespread. It is a visual representation of embracing the way a person was created. I personally like the As I Am products not only because I think the products are good but also because I love the message in the title. Ironically, hair—or the fear of messing up our hair—is one reason that women often cite for not becoming physically active. I'm not saying the struggle isn't real. It most definitely is. However, it forces us to confront a bigger issue: Can I love me as I am to get to where I want to be? Lifestyle change is extremely hard, but with God, nothing is impossible. Right, preacher?

Ministry

It's on this very note and thought that I concluded my writing for January's discussion. Yes, nothing is impossible with God. In fact, the Apostle Paul concluded and proclaimed in Philippians 4:13 (KJV), "I can do all things through Christ which strengtheneth me." This verse is very simple in reading but a bit harder in putting into practice.

Most Christians have no problem believing that the Lord is able and willing to do just what we need Him to do. However, the struggle arises when it comes to fully relying on God. That's because even the most faithful Christian often has the tendency to make God the last resort rather than the first resource. We tend to use God on an emergency basis rather than as our source and strength for everything. However, we must come to the same realization that Paul reached when he declared that our sufficiency is not in ourselves, but in God (2 Corinthians 3:5).

Why are lifestyle changes—and changes in general—so hard at times? First, the problem often lies in the desires within us. Some people, in the context of this conversation, know they're unhealthy, know they're abusing their bodies, and know they're consistently putting themselves at risk for major health problems. However, they simply don't want to quit feeding what satisfies their flesh. They rationalize their behaviors. You've heard it. Smoking soothes them. Food comforts them. And alcohol sedates them to life's problems. Unfortunately, for many people, the very things they enjoy and declare they need to just to make it are the very things contributing to their downfall and demise.

However, some people genuinely and truly want to change for the better. They've tried with modest, if any, success. After trying many times, they grow weary with trying. Then there are those whose hearts and minds say, "Let's do it." However, deep within they feel they don't have the inner energy and sustaining power to accomplish their goals.

Having struggled with weight for a few years, I know this feeling. That's why it's *so* important to have a great support group of people who are uniquely gifted to embrace others with truth and compassion. A great support structure doesn't enable you, it knows when and how to encourage you. Key supporters also know how to turn your attention from yourself to your Savior—from the beginning!

We'll talk about connections and support structures a bit later. For now, it's about asking God for strength and having some strong, truthful conversations with the man or woman in the mirror. Tell yourself: "I shall live and not die." "The battle is worth it." "I can't do this alone. But with *God*, I can. He will sustain me and see me through."

When you get to the point of the honest *mirror conversation*, coupled with friends and loved ones who love you and want to see you healthy and successful, then change will begin to happen. In most cases, the changes will happen slowly but surely. Will there be failures and setbacks? Sure. However, you must keep reminding yourself that this is truly a journey and marathon—not a quick sprint.

February

February is heart month. Let's work on having a healthy and uplifted heart. Love yourself enough to take care of yourself. What are your goals for February?

1.

2.

3.

February 1st

Thought of the Day

Who people are on Instagram often is not who they are in real life. Don't get fooled by the filters, the flossing, and the borrowed wisdom. If you start to feel inadequate because of what you see on social media, remember Instagram is never more powerful than the Great I Am. You were created to be exactly who you are. Learn when to tune out social media so you can tune in to you.

My prayer for today is:

_____

_____

_____

What I will do today to love myself:

_____

_____

_____

_____

My thoughts for today:

_____

_____

_____

_____

_____

February 2nd

Thought of the Day

I have learned lessons from my hair journey. I wore straightened hair for the longest time. My stylist would style every little hair so that not even one was out of place. When I started going natural, every hair was not always perfect. It took a while for me to accept that it was okay not being absolutely perfect. It didn't mean that my hair didn't look good. I watched videos of ladies doing a million steps to get great curls. I realized at some point that what they did was not necessarily best for me. I learned to do a few quick steps that work for me. I learned that I felt freer to exercise with my natural hair. I'm not scared of sweating or even the rain. Best of all, I learned to quiet the haters. No one can tell me the way that I was created is not good enough. With me, there's no false advertisement. You know what you are getting. For those who don't like it, they are not the right fit for me. I am authentic. I'm a natural woman with natural hair. If you don't like it, I don't care. Natural hair may not be your jam, but you can learn a lesson from natural hair. You can be perfectly imperfect and love yourself. And never forget that the God who created you in all your splendor loves you, too!

My prayer for today is:

_____

_____

_____

What I will do today to love myself:

_____

_____

_____

_____

My thoughts for today:

_____

_____

_____

_____

_____

February 3rd

Thought of the Day

God purposely created us with many insufficiencies and inadequacies to make certain our dependence is on Him. There are many things we simply can't do on our own. That's because God wants to continually remind us that we need Him and that He's near us! Fully rely on our loving Father.

My prayer for today is:

_____

_____

_____

What I will do today to love myself:

_____

_____

_____

_____

My thoughts for today:

_____

_____

_____

_____

_____

February 4th

Thought of the Day

Teddy Roosevelt said, "Nothing worth having comes easy." The same can apply to achieving a healthy lifestyle. It requires discipline. Do things like plan your menu. You may even decide to set aside time to prep all of your meals for the entire week. Put exercise on your schedule. Incorporate meditation into your plan. Treat those things as importantly as you do meetings or other commitments. It takes a significant investment, but the return on that investment will be exponentially higher.

My prayer for today is:

_____

_____

_____

What I will do today to love myself:

_____

_____

_____

_____

My thoughts for today:

_____

_____

_____

_____

_____

February 5th

Thought of the Day

The beauty of 1 Corinthians 13 is that it describes love that can be applied to romantic relationships and friendships alike. That love can exist between neighbors. It compels us to be kind to others. Sometimes it's not that we're looking for love in all the wrong places. We just don't recognize love when we see it. Love and allow yourself to be loved.

My prayer for today is:

_____

_____

_____

What I will do today to love myself:

_____

_____

_____

My thoughts for today:

_____

_____

_____

_____

February 6th

Thought of the Day

A good friend of mine said that sometimes the person I am called to be is not always the person I am. I can relate to that. There are settings where an introvert is required to be an extrovert. Sometimes a follower is called upon to be a leader. Those transitions can be extremely difficult. They take us out of our comfort zones. Just remember where your calling comes from. It will help you to convey on the outside whose you are on the inside. Embrace your calling!

My prayer for today is:

_____

_____

_____

What I will do today to love myself:

_____

_____

_____

_____

My thoughts for today:

_____

_____

_____

_____

_____

February 7th

Thought of the Day

Everybody talks about work-life balance. It's become a buzz word. It's about how you distribute your time across your priorities in a manner that lets you live a full and happy life. There's no perfect formula for it. It's different for everybody. If you are doing what you love, your work may mesh well with your life outside of work. Don't let anybody decide for you what your balance looks like. When your spirit to make a difference is consistent across both your work and your life outside of work, you may have found your balance. God will keep you in perfect peace, if your mind is stayed on Him.

My prayer for today is:

_____

_____

_____

What I will do today to love myself:

_____

_____

_____

_____

My thoughts for today:

_____

_____

_____

_____

_____

February 8th

Thought of the Day

Sometimes we make excuses for not moving ahead because we're too afraid of letting go of the past. We'll hold on to toxic relationships because we're afraid of being alone. We'll hold on to pain because it's familiar. Don't dwell in yesterday. Step out on faith today. Look forward to a brighter tomorrow.

My prayer for today is:

_____

_____

_____

What I will do today to love myself:

_____

_____

_____

_____

My thoughts for today:

_____

_____

_____

_____

_____

February 9th

Thought of the Day

We've all heard a version of the quote about insanity: insanity is doing the same thing over and over and expecting a different result. That can apply to so many things whether it's losing weight, your job, a relationship, or direction in life. Identifying the insanity is not the travesty. Staying in it is.

My prayer for today is:

_____

_____

_____

What I will do today to love myself:

_____

_____

_____

My thoughts for today:

_____

_____

_____

_____

February 10th

Thought of the Day

I've learned to not read my own press. Many good things could be said, but that one negative comment will play over and over in my mind. If I've done something positive, I get feedback in other ways so I don't have to read someone's interpretation. If I've missed the mark, I prefer to get constructive criticism from someone who knows my intent versus a cowardly troll seeking to make me feel bad. I don't focus on the press, because it doesn't write my story. I challenge you to write your story for the world to read.

My prayer for today is:

_____

_____

_____

What I will do today to love myself:

_____

_____

_____

_____

My thoughts for today:

_____

_____

_____

_____

_____

February 11th

Thought of the Day

The more you chase images of who you are not, the more you become disappointed in who you are. Media will try to tell us what is beautiful. I'm always astounded when a model is deemed beautiful because of a unique feature like a mole on the face or a gap between the two front teeth. We accept it in others, but then we look in the mirror and think our uniqueness is a flaw. We sometimes forget that beauty comes from the inside. Changing our features won't change our insecurities. Instead, we should change our mindsets. Celebrate your beauty. The mirror shouldn't be the only place you look. You are beautiful!

My prayer for today is:

_____

_____

_____

What I will do today to love myself:

_____

_____

_____

_____

My thoughts for today:

_____

_____

_____

_____

February 12th

Thought of the Day

It's okay to take the road less traveled. And sometimes, there's the road only meant for you to travel. While it may seem a little scary, the very fact that it is a road says that your path has been cleared. As long as you have the One who is able to keep you from falling and who orders your steps, by faith you will make it to your destination.

My prayer for today is:

_____

_____

_____

What I will do today to love myself:

_____

_____

_____

_____

My thoughts for today:

_____

_____

_____

_____

_____

February 13th

Thought of the Day

I think the biggest mistake new runners make when they run their first race is that they get excited with all the others around them, and when the horn sounds, they start off running too fast. They run a pace faster than they practiced and faster than they can sustain. I was guilty of this, but I have learned to run my own pace no matter what others are doing around me. Some of the people who left me in the dust at the start line looked at my back when I crossed the finish line. The Bible says, "The race is not to the swift" (Ecclesiastes 9:11, KJV). My friends, go out and run your race!

My prayer for today is:

_____

_____

_____

What I will do today to love myself:

_____

_____

_____

_____

My thoughts for today:

_____

_____

_____

_____

_____

February 14th

Thought of the Day

An anonymous individual said, "It takes a strong person to remain single in a world that is accustomed to settling with anything just to say they have something." Celebrate your strengths if you are single. Know your worth whether you are single or in a relationship. It should not be up for negotiation.

My prayer for today is:

_____

_____

_____

What I will do today to love myself:

_____

_____

_____

_____

My thoughts for today:

_____

_____

_____

_____

_____

February 15th

Thought of the Day

One of my friends went to a counseling session. The counselor started by asking, "Are you willing to be made willing?" In other words, are your heart and mind open to change and compromise? Change does not happen unless you are ready to submit to it. Friends, are you willing to be made willing?

My prayer for today is:

_____

_____

_____

What I will do today to love myself:

_____

_____

_____

_____

My thoughts for today:

_____

_____

_____

_____

_____

February 16th

Thought of the Day

You don't need everyone to agree with you, be with you, like you, or understand you as long as you are completely confident that you are the "you" that God intends for you to be. God will always be to you what others can never be. He'll always do what no other person can do. By all means, we should seek fruitful relationships with others. But first, make sure that you have a relationship with God.

My prayer for today is:

_____

_____

_____

What I will do today to love myself:

_____

_____

_____

_____

My thoughts for today:

_____

_____

_____

_____

_____

February 17th

Thought of the Day

Don't fret every imperfection and everything that you deem is wrong in your life. Instead, just keep striving to be better and to do better each day. Always keep in mind that you're not a finished product yet. God is still fixing, forming, and favoring you. So focus, go forward, and let the Father do what He does!

My prayer for today is:

_____

_____

_____

What I will do today to love myself:

_____

_____

_____

_____

My thoughts for today:

_____

_____

_____

_____

_____

February 18th

Thought of the Day

If you have to beg others to be committed to anything or anyone, rest assured they're not committed at all. Instead, they're temporarily conforming just to quiet you, to ease pressure, or to continue on their own personal project. Commitment doesn't require constant badgering!

My prayer for today is:

_____

_____

_____

What I will do today to love myself:

_____

_____

_____

_____

My thoughts for today:

_____

_____

_____

_____

_____

February 19th

Thought of the Day

Andy Rooney once said, "If you smile when you are alone, you really mean it." Have you watched someone taking a selfie and you think, "That smile is so fake." Today, too many people are posing for the camera or others. When you have true joy, the smile that shows on the outside radiates from the inside. It doesn't require "likes" to be validated.

My prayer for today is:

_____

_____

_____

What I will do today to love myself:

_____

_____

_____

_____

My thoughts for today:

_____

_____

_____

_____

_____

February 20th

Thought of the Day

Sometimes it helps to set a goal to work toward. It's cool to want to fit in a favorite dress or outfit. Even more motivating is choosing a goal that focuses on something bigger. For example, consider doing a 5K for charity. The goal is to benefit others, but a great side effect of your training is that you will get in better shape. The feeling you get when you cross the finish line may just be enough to inspire you to do another 5k or even a 10k. Strengthening your heart may bless someone else's!

My prayer for today is:

_____

_____

_____

What I will do today to love myself:

_____

_____

_____

_____

My thoughts for today:

_____

_____

_____

_____

_____

February 21st

Thought of the Day

Muhammad Ali said, "I am the greatest. I said that even before I knew I was." He expressed it as only Muhammed Ali could. The message is that sometimes you have to proclaim a thing over your life and walk into it. The Bible says, "Now faith is the substance of things hoped for and the evidence of things not seen" (Hebrews 11:1, KJV). Be great!

My prayer for today is:

_____

_____

_____

What I will do today to love myself:

_____

_____

_____

My thoughts for today:

_____

_____

_____

_____

February 22nd

Thought of the Day

Nowadays, people will journal on social media. They share their sorrows, joys, and even journeys they're about to embark on. If that's done for accountability, that could be one way of achieving that. The problem is when things take a negative turn based on a low number of likes or if negative comments enter the feed. One negative comment can linger and outweigh all the positive ones. Consider making your journey more private. It is your journey. Galatians 1:10 (NIV) says, "Am I now trying to win the approval of human beings, or of God? Or am I still trying to please people, I would not be a servant of Christ."

My prayer for today is:

_____

_____

_____

What I will do today to love myself:

_____

_____

_____

_____

My thoughts for today:

_____

_____

_____

_____

February 23rd

Thought of the Day

Your worth and value are not determined by someone else's appraisal of you. Rather, worth and value are established by your relationship with God and your living out HIS purpose for your life. Make it a blessed day!

My prayer for today is:

_____

_____

_____

What I will do today to love myself:

_____

_____

_____

_____

My thoughts for today:

_____

_____

_____

_____

February 24th

Thought of the Day

Yes, we are to help "bear the infirmities of the weak" (Romans 15:1, KJV). However, the Bible never tells us to be broken by the infirmities and issues of others. If one's not careful, one will still be reeling over someone else's problem while that person has gone on to the next thing in his or her life. Do what you can to help others; but learn your limits. Learn when and how to leave them in the hands of the Lord. Take care of yourself on this blessed day!

My prayer for today is:

_____

_____

_____

What I will do today to love myself:

_____

_____

_____

_____

My thoughts for today:

_____

_____

_____

_____

_____

February 25th

Thought of the Day

Most half marathons and marathons offer parties at the end. They usually include food, beverages, and music. It's so much fun to see sweaty people with medals draped around their necks having such a good time. I admit that I have to take a pic of myself, salty face and all, to send to family and close friends. Maybe it's not the prettiest picture, but I feel absolutely beautiful. I am grateful to God for allowing me to run my race and finish. The glow from gratitude is better than any makeup I could ever buy!

My prayer for today is:

_____

_____

_____

What I will do today to love myself:

_____

_____

_____

_____

My thoughts for today:

_____

_____

_____

_____

_____

February 26th

Thought of the Day

The song *It is For Me* has a line that says, "What God has for me, it is for me." Don't wish for what others have or appear to have. Besides, you don't know what they've been through before they realized their blessing. Jeremiah 29:11 (NIV) says, "'For I know the plans I have for you,' declares the Lord, 'plans to prosper you and not to harm you, plans to give you a hope and a future.'" Spend your time preparing your body, mind, and spirit for what is uniquely ordained to come your way!

My prayer for today is:

_____

_____

_____

What I will do today to love myself:

_____

_____

_____

_____

My thoughts for today:

_____

_____

_____

_____

February 27th

Thought of the Day

A friend of mine is battling breast cancer. When asked about her support system, she talks affectionately about her birth family and her chosen family. She shares blood with her birth family. With her chosen family, there is a strong bond that binds like blood. God gives you what you need in a variety of places. Don't get so focused on looking for love in just one place. It might be all around you.

My prayer for today is:

_____

_____

_____

What I will do today to love myself:

_____

_____

_____

_____

My thoughts for today:

_____

_____

_____

_____

_____

February 28th

Thought of the Day

Today, simply resolve to be the very best version of yourself. That means fully embracing who you are right now and being excited about who God is developing you to be in the future. At day's end, celebrate the fact that you're unique, and there is no one else anywhere like the masterpiece called YOU! Now be you and do you on this FABULOUS day

My prayer for today is:

_____

_____

_____

What I will do today to love myself:

_____

_____

_____

_____

My thoughts for today:

_____

_____

_____

_____

_____

February 29th (or bonus):

Thought of the Day

It is a great thing to be able to forgive because it is liberating for you. It allows you to move on. However, you can forgive while not forfeiting your rights for justice or demanding better treatment if you've been wronged. Forgiveness should be the compassion that fuels the passion to see right prevail.

My prayer for today is:

_____

_____

_____

What I will do today to love myself:

_____

_____

_____

My thoughts for today:

_____

_____

_____

_____

March

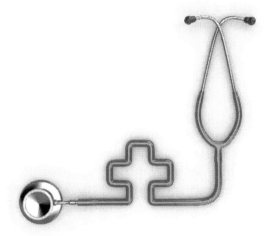

March
Madness or Gladness?

Medicine

If you are a college basketball fan, you know that all roads lead to March Madness! It is the big college tournament that ultimately determines the best team in the nation. It is very exciting. The energy is palpable. One of the things that we all wait for is who will emerge as the Cinderella team—the team that not many people have noticed. They seem to come out of nowhere. Even though they appear on the bracket, no one pays them any attention. They are counted out before they ever hit the court.

I wonder what it's like for them in the locker room. I imagine them rallying around their collective belief that they possess the talent, the work ethic, the heart, and the mindset to be victorious. I can see them with heads bowed during a team prayer before heading out to the court. I can hear the coach saying, "Keep your heads in the game. No matter what, let's play our game." They hear the crowd cheering for the other team as they wait in the wings. They notice the lack of cheers and even hear some boos as they exit the tunnel to take the floor. None of those negative seeds plant in their minds. They are focused. Tip-off occurs. They stumble through the first few plays. The coach calls a time out and reminds them to focus. As their minds settle, their talent and teamwork show up. They silence the boos. Before you know it, the crowd can't deny their skill and determination and cheer them on. In that moment, they know they can go all the way.

I believe that a significant number of people in the church have mental health issues who don't feel like they can suit up and get in the game. They sit on the bench because they think they are alone. There are spectators, some real and some perceived, signaling for them to quietly stay out of the game for fear of embarrassment. They may even have a spiritual coach or two telling them to simply pray their mental health issues away. I don't know of any basketball player who has gotten better by sitting on the bench. I don't know of any basketball superstars who haven't referenced a coach who helped them to cultivate their strengths and to build up their deficits in order to get better.

What if the church were an advocate for mental health? What if they cheered the Cinderella hopeful on? It is not unlike physical health in that there are conditions that are treatable. Getting help doesn't replace faith. It augments it. Churches widely vary on where they stand on mental health. I hope that embracing mental health wellness becomes the norm. We can't be afraid to talk about mental health in the church. The Bible says, "For God has not given us the spirit of fear, but of power, and of love, and of a sound mind" (2 Timothy 1:7, KJV). Right, preacher?

Ministry

First, let me say that *praying away* some problems, issues, and concerns is a very valid thing to do. There are a ton of examples in the Bible where faith-filled, powerful, and persistent prayer was the catalyst for the deliverance people needed. Prayer is a game-changer. Prayer is a spiritual change agent.

That said, it's a fact that some simply "wait on God to move" and do little else. I'm a firm believer that there is no need for the supernatural until first we've exhausted everything spiritual, logical, and reasonable in our natural. In the case of mental health, while believing God and waiting on Him to move on our behalf, we can and should embrace the fact that He's already provided help among us with many Spirit-filled, trained professionals who can address issues and place us on a path of mental healing and wholeness. More on this later as well.

As for the church addressing mental issues, I agree that churches must venture beyond just having good worship experiences and truly minister to their congregants in a more holistic manner. However, let's not paint a picture of gross negligence on the church for maybe not being the greatest advocate for mental health. I firmly believe that there are many pastors and churches that don't address it consistently and intentionally for a couple of reasons.

First, having a wide circle of friends who are pastors, I know that mental health is a conversation that rarely comes up among pastors. It's just not a part of the fodder. I think that largely has to do with there not being a great understanding among church leadership *and* laity about what mental health really is. Just the two words *mental illness* quickly imply to many people that someone is *crazy*. However, we know that mental health covers a wide gamut of ailments, conditions, and presentations.

Second, not only do many people not really understand what mental health wellness means or the depths of what mental illness encompasses, I'm convinced that many church leaders don't recognize the prevalence of the presence of mental health issues within their congregations. There may be one or two we deem as *obvious* cases. Still, to the untrained eye, what does depression really look like? What does a dangerously low self-esteem look or sound like? How do I recognize anxieties or eating disorders? What are signs of addiction? My stained-glass view may not show me these things. Therefore, how can the church address what, in many cases, it's ignorant of?

I think this is where ministry and medicine really must meet. Passionate people from both of these arenas must come to the table and have a true discourse about mental health. Medical professionals must make it plain what we're dealing with daily regarding mental health and mental illness. Ministry leaders must embrace the fact that we and our churches are needed to help *coach* and encourage our congregants so they'll see subtle, yet steady improvement in their lives. The same faith that we believe produces favorable results in our physical health is the same faith we believe will prevail in mental health. It's just in most cases, there must be real conversations about mental health before there can be convictions and commitments from the church to tackle it head on.

Have you done this for your church? If so, how? And what has been the impact? What's the call to action for me as an individual and not as the clergy who need to take the lead?

March

Our hope this month is that by faith you will confront anxieties, depression, or anything that challenges your inner peace. We also pray that you will seek help for mental wellness if you need it. Make a declaration that you WILL be glad! What are your goals for March?

1.

2.

3.

March 1st

Thought of the Day

When I was a child, I remember that often during the devotional period, some of the more seasoned people in the church would pray and thank God for their being "clothed in their right minds." In other words, they thanked God for being mentally intact. Witnesses to that prayer would signal agreement by saying, "Amen." Let's extend that prayer to those needing help to become mentally whole. Let us not be ashamed if we are the ones in need. Corporately, we can take away the stigma surrounding mental health. A diagnosis doesn't define you. Asking for help is not a sign of weakness—it's a strong step in the right direction.

My prayer for today is:

_____

_____

_____

What I will do today to be glad:

_____

_____

_____

My thoughts for today:

_____

_____

_____

_____

March 2nd

Thought of the Day

Sometimes the best blessings are following by experiences we just can't explain. For example, some women have babies and shortly thereafter develop postpartum depression. It can be hard to admit because they truly are ecstatic over the birth of their babies but the hormonal surge leaves them feeling off balance. Others of us have what we would call mountain-top experiences and then we crash into a valley and we don't understand why. We all cry sometimes but know when we need to cry out for help. Prayer can change things. Sometimes those prayers need to include asking God when we need to seek help from someone He has ordained to do that. Those people are extensions of His love—not a contradiction of it. Don't suffer in silence!

My prayer for today is:

_____

_____

_____

What I will do today to be glad:

_____

_____

_____

_____

My thoughts for today:

_____

_____

_____

_____

_____

March 3rd

Thought of the Day

The value of a strong, made-up mind is that you learn not to mind others who have no mind to do the right things and to excel. Those same people may try to make you and others believe that you've lost your mind because you won't condescend to mediocrity and accept just anything. Little do they know that your heart is fixed and your mind is made up that you're going to be successful and do things the right way. All the while, you'll give God glory and make those around you better. So friend, keep your mind on the business at hand and conquer your day!

My prayer for today is:

_____

_____

_____

What I will do today to be glad:

_____

_____

_____

_____

My thoughts for today:

_____

_____

_____

_____

_____

March 4th

Thought of the Day

We've heard the saying so many times: "I'm not getting old. I'm getting better." There is something so liberating when you understand that getting older doesn't mean you to have to get old. Each year after winter loosens its grip, spring shows up with its golden sun. I, like many others, bask in the warmth and marvel at the flowers blooming and the trees turning green. Although it happens every year, it never gets old. It just ushers in a new season. Each day, we have new grace and new mercies. Embrace changes in life and celebrate your seasons!

My prayer for today is:

_____

_____

_____

What I will do today to be glad:

_____

_____

_____

_____

My thoughts for today:

_____

_____

_____

_____

_____

March 5th

Thought of the Day

It's so easy for us to react versus respond. A reaction is quick and not well thought out. It tends to elicit a less than favorable reaction from the person with whom we are interacting. It doesn't usually lead to a constructive outcome. A response is slower and better thought out. It allows for reason. Start practicing James 1:19 (NIV), "My dear brothers and sisters, take note of this. Everyone should be quick to listen, slow to speak, and slow to become angry." Today, practice letting your response reflect whose child you are.

My prayer for today is:

_____

_____

_____

What I will do today to be glad:

_____

_____

_____

_____

My thoughts for today:

_____

_____

_____

_____

_____

March 6th

Thought of the Day

Father, thanks so much for another day. Help me through every stressful situation. Please hear my prayers and let me be sensitive to your Spirit so that I can feel Your presence, Your power, Your love, and Your compassion. Please let me not be ashamed to seek help from those you have ordained to give me prudent counsel for my life. I ask these things in the powerful name of Jesus.

My prayer for today is:

_____

_____

_____

What I will do today to be glad:

_____

_____

_____

_____

My thoughts for today:

_____

_____

_____

_____

_____

March 7th

Thought of the Day

I love what Theodore Roosevelt said: "The credit belongs to the man who is actually in the arena, whose face is marred by dust and sweat and blood, who knows the great enthusiasms, the great devotions, and spends himself in a worthy cause; who at best, if he wins, knows the thrills of high achievement, and, if he fails, at least fails daring greatly, so that his place shall never be with those cold and timid souls who know neither victory nor defeat." You can't expect to win if you never get in the game.

My prayer for today is:

_____

_____

_____

What I will do today to be glad:

_____

_____

_____

_____

My thoughts for today:

_____

_____

_____

_____

_____

March 8th

Thought of the Day

People are often not sure if they are dealing with depression. It can be hard to know. Here are a few questions to ask yourself. Is my sad mood persistent? Have I lost interest in things I use to enjoy? Am I having trouble falling asleep or staying asleep regularly? Do I sleep too much? Is my energy gone? If you answer yes to several of these, it may be time to have a conversation with your primary care provider. It's time for you to say yes to a brighter day for you.

My prayer for today is:

_____

_____

_____

What I will do today to be glad:

_____

_____

_____

My thoughts for today:

_____

_____

_____

_____

_____

March 9th

Thought of the Day

It is hard to not be affected by our current environment. There are too many reports of shootings these days and other cruel injustices toward human beings. Let's face it. These things are depressing. It makes me want to turn off the TV and radio because I can't hardly stand hearing about it anymore. I have decided that I have to channel those feelings of despondence into energy to make a positive difference. I've run an 8K to support the families of a shooting incident. It won't bring their love ones back, but seeing those families reminded me that I can do even more. I can vote and encourage others to vote to change the system. Even though change takes a while, it doesn't mean we don't make the effort and keep making the effort. Be a part of the change you want to see for yourself and for others.

My prayer for today is:

_____

_____

_____

What I will do today to be glad:

_____

_____

_____

_____

My thoughts for today:

_____

_____

_____

_____

_____

March 10th

Thought of the Day

Peace doesn't necessarily diffuse every storm cloud. However, it does give you a faith vision to be able to peer through the clouds and see the sun shining in the future. No matter what the eyes see, peace lets your heart know that things are going to be okay. Walk in peace today.

My prayer for today is:

_____

_____

_____

What I will do today to be glad:

_____

_____

_____

My thoughts for today:

_____

_____

_____

_____

March 11th

Thought of the Day

We need to stop and celebrate the things we sometimes take for granted. Thanking God for peace of mind is a great start! So many people are homeless because a mental condition controls their world. Many people have become addicted to alcohol and drugs as a result of struggling with emotional issues. Every day that we wake up with a mind that is focused enough for us to assess if we're okay is a huge blessing. If that assessment leads us to seek help, we should ask God for the strength to pursue it. Not dealing with our issues can escalate into situations that can become a bigger struggle. If you are asking yourself if you're okay, you might need counsel to help you objectively answer that question. Pursue clarity from any confusion you might have in your life.

My prayer for today is:

_____

_____

_____

What I will do today to be glad:

_____

_____

_____

_____

My thoughts for today:

_____

_____

_____

_____

_____

March 12th

Thought of the Day

Your future is way too bright for you to sulk and become stagnant because of a couple of miscues and missed opportunities. Pick yourself up. Dust yourself off. Raise your head. Quicken your heart and spirit. Do God. Do you. Then do greater things than you ever have before. There is too much ahead for you to bury your head where you are now.

My prayer for today is:

_____

_____

_____

What I will do today to be glad:

_____

_____

_____

_____

My thoughts for today:

_____

_____

_____

_____

_____

March 13th

Thought of the Day

I remember hearing the story about a man who was in an area where a big flood was predicted to come. Officials came around in a car to try to get him to evacuate. He declined to go saying, "God will take care of me." The flood began. The next time officials came to try to evacuate him, they had to come in a boat. He refused to evacuate then, too, saying, "God will take care of me." The water kept rising. The man had to get on his roof. Officials came in a helicopter to rescue him. He refused to go with them saying, "God will take care of me." The flood overcame him. When he got to heaven, he asked God why He didn't save him. He had told everybody, "God will take care of me." God said, "I sent a car, a boat, and a helicopter." Don't miss God's help for your life because you have your mind set that help can only come in one way.

My prayer for today is:

_____

_____

_____

What I will do today to be glad:

_____

_____

_____

_____

My thoughts for today:

_____

_____

_____

_____

_____

March 14th

Thought of the Day

If you fill yourself seeking after the heart of God, and the Word of God as the mode of operation and the motivation for your life, there should be no room left within you to lean to your own understanding (Proverbs 3:5-6) or to feed and follow your flesh. It's simple. Either you lean on Him or you lean on yourself. Each person must make that choice for himself or herself. Take the time to glorify God on this MARVELOUS day.

My prayer for today is:

_____

_____

_____

What I will do today to be glad:

_____

_____

_____

_____

My thoughts for today:

_____

_____

_____

_____

_____

March 15th

Thought of the Day

Sometimes people will misinterpret your kindness for weakness. Don't let their miscalculation of you change your demeanor. Use it to your advantage. The power of your self-control speaks loudly without you even raising your voice. Walk calmly into victory!

My prayer for today is:

_____

_____

_____

What I will do today to be glad:

_____

_____

_____

_____

My thoughts for today:

_____

_____

_____

_____

_____

March 16th

Thought of the Day

I think one of the greatest beauties of science is that it studies and appreciates the miracles of God. Take something like a joint replacement for example. While it uses materials made by man, it recreates the natural motion of the joint and often alleviates pain. Resident doctors in training are taught by more experienced attending physicians. I believe physicians and counselors called by God never stray away from the ultimate creator and healer. Don't be afraid to seek help from one of God's children that has taken up the family business of healing.

My prayer for today is:

_____

_____

_____

What I will do today to be glad:

_____

_____

_____

_____

My thoughts for today:

_____

_____

_____

_____

_____

March 17th

Thought of the Day

Believe in yourself enough that you can see yourself in the winner's circle before the starting gun is even shot. A third of winning is a mindset that believes. A third of winning is determination. A third of winning is execution. You got this!

My prayer for today is:

_____

_____

_____

What I will do today to be glad:

_____

_____

_____

_____

My thoughts for today:

_____

_____

_____

_____

_____

March 18th

Thought of the Day

I've learned in life that many times when we think we need a miracle, all we really need is a made-up mind. I'm a firm believer that God can do and does do many things supernaturally. However, oftentimes the supernatural is not needed if we would just make up our minds to handle our business in the natural. Put even simpler, do your very best and THEN see God do the rest.

My prayer for today is:

_____

_____

_____

What I will do today to be glad:

_____

_____

_____

My thoughts for today:

_____

_____

_____

_____

_____

March 19th

Thought of the Day

The journey on your way to where you're going is most often shaped by the experiences, failures, and triumphs of where you've been and also by an honest, accurate assessment of where you are right now. Live. Learn. Keep it real. Let's have a favored day.

My prayer for today is:

_____

_____

_____

What I will do today to be glad:

_____

_____

_____

_____

My thoughts for today:

_____

_____

_____

_____

_____

March 20th

Thought of the Day

One of the things I love to see is a glimpse of heaven on earth. Sam Cooke sang a song that said it well: "A little flower that blooms in May. A lovely sunset at the end of a day. Someone helping a stranger along the way. That's heaven to me." Don't get so caught up wondering if God is up there. Take time to see that He is everywhere.

My prayer for today is:

_____

_____

_____

What I will do today to be glad:

_____

_____

_____

_____

My thoughts for today:

_____

_____

_____

_____

_____

March 21st

Thought of the Day

I often borrow these lyrics from Donny Hathaway, "If my words don't come together, listen to my melody." I try really hard for people to know my heart and my character. So when those days come when I don't always know the right thing to say, my actions and my track record still speak my truth. No auto-tuning is needed. My character has established my true voice. Go out and write a melody today.

My prayer for today is:

_____

_____

_____

What I will do today to be glad:

_____

_____

_____

_____

My thoughts for today:

_____

_____

_____

_____

_____

March 22nd

Thought of the Day

For the believer, it's never luck; it's always the Lord. In our minds, it's never just "all good"; but we forever declare that every blessing, every healing, every provision, every miracle, every open door, and every opportunity is "ALL GOD!"

My prayer for today is:

_____

_____

_____

What I will do today to be glad:

_____

_____

_____

My thoughts for today:

_____

_____

_____

_____

March 23rd

Thought of the Day

Sometimes you have to learn how to encourage yourself in the Lord and to speak life, health, strength, provision, protection, and blessings over YOUR OWN LIFE. To do so engages the faith and focus needed to carry you through just about anything.

My prayer for today is:

_____

_____

_____

What I will do today to be glad:

_____

_____

_____

_____

My thoughts for today:

_____

_____

_____

_____

_____

March 24th

Thought of the Day

The tragedy that many people endure is that they're defeated the moment they start thinking. What you think about yourself and where you see yourself are great indicators of what will eventually be your reality. Friend, you have "the pen" to write your own narrative. The question is, will your mindset today cause you to write your continually evolving story or are you set on quitting and writing your obituary? You're the author. You decide!

My prayer for today is:

_____

_____

_____

What I will do today to be glad:

_____

_____

_____

_____

My thoughts for today:

_____

_____

_____

_____

_____

March 25th

Thought of the Day

Sometimes you just have to press, pray, and praise your way through. But the one thing you can't do is give up now! Watch God work on this WONDERFUL day.

My prayer for today is:

_____

_____

_____

What I will do today to be glad:

_____

_____

_____

_____

My thoughts for today:

_____

_____

_____

_____

March 26th

Thought of the Day

The big chop. That's all I have to say for naturalistas to know what I'm talking about. So, if you had been getting chemicals in your hair to make it straight and now you want to go with your natural curls, it is likely you'll need to go for the big chop! The big chop is a haircut that cuts away all of your straightened hair, leaving just the hair closest to your scalp that has its natural curl pattern and hasn't been straightened by chemicals. That can be so hard for those parting with lots of hair that took years to grow! We can try to avoid it and just get the ends cut. You end up with curly hair at the roots and straight hair at the ends. Every time you pass the mirror, you know you need the big chop. When you finally do it, you are left with strong, beautiful hair that has not been processed. It will start to grow and show your real pattern. Sometimes we need to do a big chop in our lives. Everybody surrounding you is not trying to go where you are. They are comfortable in their complacency. Others in your life may hinder your progress. Make up your mind to do the big chop. Your beautiful growth awaits.

My prayer for today is:

_____

_____

_____

What I will do today to be glad:

_____

_____

_____

_____

My thoughts for today:

_____

_____

_____

_____

_____

March 27th

Thought of the Day

Living to prove your worth to someone isn't living—it's bondage. Instead, live the way God intends for you to live. Then your worth and potential will be displayed undeniably. You need no one to validate you since God has already established you. Approach this day knowing your value.

My prayer for today is:

_____

_____

_____

What I will do today to be glad:

_____

_____

_____

_____

My thoughts for today:

_____

_____

_____

_____

_____

March 28th

Thought of the Day

If you prayed about it in faith, there is no need to panic, grow weary, and faint about it! Trust the God you told about it!

My prayer for today is:

_____

_____

_____

What I will do today to be glad:

_____

_____

_____

_____

My thoughts for today:

_____

_____

_____

_____

_____

March 29th

Thought of the Day

True friends are easily identified. These are the people who are closest to you when you have legitimate needs and little to offer them in return. True friends are the ones there when you're enduring as the victim and not just there for the victory party when the trouble ends. Thank God for true friends. By the way, be reminded that the GREATEST friend of all is Jesus Christ.

My prayer for today is:

_____

_____

_____

What I will do today to be glad:

_____

_____

_____

My thoughts for today:

_____

_____

_____

_____

March 30th

Thought of the Day

God created you. Therefore, trust Him to sustain and steer your life. Live confidently knowing that God cares for and keeps everything and everyone He created. Don't dishonor Him by wondering if you are good enough. It took years for Michelangelo to paint the ceiling of the Sistine Chapel. It also took years for Leonardo da Vinci to paint the Mona Lisa. They are both regarded as masterpieces. Just because God still has His paintbrush on you doesn't mean you aren't a masterpiece. Walk in your beauty.

My prayer for today is:

_____

_____

_____

What I will do today to be glad:

_____

_____

_____

_____

My thoughts for today:

_____

_____

_____

_____

_____

March 31st

Thought of the Day

If God hasn't said it's over, keep the faith, keep fighting, keep believing, and keep working. One thing is certain, if you quit now you won't know what could have been. You won't realize your goal and receive the blessings tied to it. Others who may have been blessed by what you could have accomplished will be impacted as well. Don't block your blessings or someone else's. Continue to fight with faith.

My prayer for today is:

_____

_____

_____

What I will do today to be glad:

_____

_____

_____

_____

My thoughts for today:

_____

_____

_____

_____

April

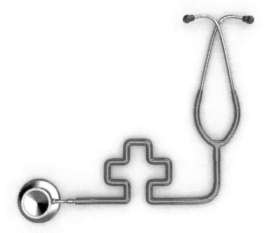

April
He Rose, but Did We?

Medicine

Easter Sunday! Resurrection Sunday! There's nothing like it. The churches are full on that day. Everyone is in his or her Sunday best. Pastel colors are in full bloom. Little girls are wearing pretty dresses and displaying perfectly styled hair. Little boys transform into little men in suits. Stomachs are rumbling at the thought of the big brunches that wait after church. Everyone listens intently as the preacher tells the familiar story of how Jesus died on the cross for our sins and how He rose *right* early on the morning of the third day with all power in His hands.

The story goes on to say that He gave us the gift of that power. Do we use that gift to the fullest extent? Do we even use it all? Do we use that power to help our fellow man? Do we liberate our families? Do we use that power to better ourselves and the world around us? The beauty of the resurrection is that we are healed because of it. We tend to only apply that healing to the well-being of our souls. What about being well in body, mind, and spirit?

In the medical world, *silent killers* refers to complications of diseases that go largely unnoticed until they become so severe that they can no longer go unnoticed. It means that damage is occurring internally within the body. If left unaddressed, these worsening conditions lead to damage that can't be reversed. Both diabetes and high blood pressure have silent killer characteristics about them. Eyesight slowly deteriorates. Kidneys slowly are compromised. Too often we pretend that if we ignore a condition, it won't really exist. Or, if we can take medication for a condition, we don't have to take personal responsibility for our lifestyles.

I believe when Jesus bestowed His power on us, it did not exclude the willpower to treat our bodies as temples. As we vow to live better lives on the heels of the resurrection, can we extend that to living healthier lives? Are we not living sacrifices, preacher?

Ministry

Yes, we are. At least that's what we are called to be. In Romans 12:1, Paul admonished us to present our bodies to God as "living sacrifices, holy, acceptable unto God which is your reasonable service." So often within the church there is great emphasis put on the gifts and talents of preaching, teaching, singing, and other things that compose and present to us what we call "having church." However, the essence of our whole existence and why God created us lies in two very basic areas. One, we are to glorify God in in our bodies. Two, we are to change the lives of those around us. These two areas extend beyond the parameters of having great church once a week. God called *all of us* into His ministry. No, you may not have (or desire) the *title* of minister. However, we all have the *task* of ministry.

What does this have to do with presenting our bodies as living sacrifices to God? Simple. If we are unhealthy physically, it's very hard to effectively and efficiently give ourselves to ministry. Let's think about it for a moment just within the context of our weekly worship experiences. How can you usher, if you can't stand for long? How can preachers minister in power if obesity or lung disease renders them breathless after 5 minutes? How can choir members sing beautifully if chemicals or other substances have damaged their vocal cords? How can dancers minister gracefully, yet powerfully, if their feet have not been properly cared for? You get the picture. If we don't care for our physical bodies, we can severely limit our effectiveness in ministry.

However, it goes deeper than that. In 1 Corinthians 6:19-20, Paul said that our bodies serve as the temple of the Holy Ghost, and we are to "glorify God in your body, and in your spirit, which are God's." At day's end, the body of the believer houses the Holy Spirit. We are to bring God glory while in this earthly body. However, we often run past the last three words of this text: "which are God's." This earthly body doesn't belong to us. This body is *on loan* to us while we breathe. Our parents taught us to take care of things that other people are kind enough to let you borrow. That principle is applicable when it comes to our bodies, too. We must ask God to bestow the power and discipline upon us to take care of our *holy houses*—our bodies.

April

Our hope for you this month is that you feel empowered to go to the next level in your life. You were given the gift of power. How will you use it? What are your goals this month?

1.

2.

3.

April 1st

Thought of the Day

I'm sure I'm like lots of you—I depend on GPS when I'm driving to places with which I'm not very familiar. Sometimes I hit start, but the GPS doesn't say anything. I know I can't just sit there so I'll start driving. I'll talk to the GPS and ask, "Are you going to say anything?" Just when I'm wondering if it's working, the voice comes on and says, "Turn right in 500 feet." Sometimes it's like that in life. You have to go in the direction you think is right. Just because it seems God is quiet doesn't mean He isn't watching. He guides you just when you were about to take a wrong turn. Don't stand still wondering which way to go. Get started on your journey, and believe God will direct your path.

My prayer for today is:

_____

_____

_____

What I will do today to exercise power in my life:

_____

_____

_____

My thoughts for today:

_____

_____

_____

_____

April 2nd

Thought of the Day

Our mother had a serious health issue that left her hospitalized. I knew when visiting her in the hospital in Alabama that I needed to move from DC and get closer to home. I had put my curriculum vitae out in Nashville just a few weeks earlier. When I returned to my house in DC from Alabama, the phone rang. I was asked to come for an interview in Nashville. I was screaming with joy. I told a friend who asked me about the position I was so excited about. I had to admit that I had no idea. When the friend asked why I was so excited, I replied, "I got on a plane, said a prayer, and the phone rang." I was interviewed a couple of weeks later. The interview was 3 hours! At the end of it, I still didn't know what the job was. What I did know was that I got on a plane, said a prayer, and the phone rang. I was offered an amazing position a few weeks later. I took it and never turned back. I got on a plane, said a prayer, and the phone rang. Step out on faith and answer your call!

My prayer for today is:

_____

_____

_____

What I will do today to exercise power in my life:

_____

_____

_____

My thoughts for today:

_____

_____

_____

_____

April 3rd

Thought of the Day

A simple word of encouragement today. Believe me when I tell you this. When it comes to what God has for you, nothing and no one can block it or stop it from coming into your life! Just remain strong and focused. Keep pressing and progressing. Most of all, stay ready to receive from God.

My prayer for today is:

_____

_____

_____

What I will do today to exercise power in my life:

_____

_____

_____

My thoughts for today:

_____

_____

_____

_____

April 4th

Thought of the Day

Michael Jordan said, "I've failed over and over and over again in my life. And that is why I succeed." Failure is not a bad thing. Defeat only comes when we don't will ourselves to get up from it. We get knocked down sometimes in life. I refuse to be counted out on a TKO. I have got to fight the good fight. Much is said about a win, but there is also victory in the fight. Fight!

My prayer for today is:

_____

_____

_____

What I will do today to exercise power in my life:

_____

_____

_____

_____

My thoughts for today:

_____

_____

_____

_____

_____

April 5th

Thought of the Day

When we honor God, our Father continually honors us. Much of what we see Him do in our lives is a direct result of us unashamedly telling Him and others who He is to us. It's called worship. In whatever capacity I worship Him, I can fully expect, by faith, for Him to work on my behalf in that capacity. For example, my heart says He's Jehovah Jireh, my Provider! So I fully expect Him to provide every one of my needs and even many of my wants and desires. Friend, brag on God. Tell Him and everybody else who He is to you. Then watch and see what He does.

My prayer for today is:

_____

_____

_____

What I will do today to exercise power in my life:

_____

_____

_____

_____

My thoughts for today:

_____

_____

_____

_____

_____

April 6th

Thought of the Day

Sometimes we get frozen in place staring at the enormous task or challenge in front of us. The mountain doesn't get smaller just because we're staring. Confucius said, "The one that moves the mountain beings by carrying away small stones." There is no time like the present to start moving stones.

My prayer for today is:

_____

_____

_____

What I will do today to exercise power in my life:

_____

_____

_____

My thoughts for today:

_____

_____

_____

_____

_____

April 7th

Thought of the Day

Sometimes you just have to press, pray, and praise your way through. But the one thing you can't do is give up now! Just because you have battle scars doesn't mean you can't win the fight. Watch God work on your behalf today.

My prayer for today is:

_____

_____

_____

What I will do today to exercise power in my life:

_____

_____

_____

_____

My thoughts for today:

_____

_____

_____

_____

_____

April 8th

Thought of the Day

Sometimes God allows our weaknesses to be glaringly obvious just so His strength will be just as obvious to us and everyone else. Even better news is that His strength will always see us through! His strength gives us power.

My prayer for today is:

_____

_____

_____

What I will do today to exercise power in my life:

_____

_____

_____

_____

My thoughts for today:

_____

_____

_____

_____

April 9th

Thought of the Day

If your course is always changed by others' opinions, it indicates that you aren't very confident or comfortable about where you're headed. Let God be your GPS. Even if you are off track right now, He will redirect you. Trust where God has you headed and stay true to that heavenly route.

My prayer for today is:

_____

_____

_____

What I will do today to exercise power in my life:

_____

_____

_____

_____

My thoughts for today:

_____

_____

_____

_____

April 10ᵗʰ

Thought of the Day

When my son was a toddler and did something that required punishment, I would ask him if he understood why he was being punished. He would say, "Yes, but I cannot like it." Sometimes life teaches us lessons that we "cannot like" but we should love the lessons that we learn. Let your mistakes make you better. I'm pretty sure you'll like that.

My prayer for today is:

_____

_____

_____

What I will do today to exercise power in my life:

_____

_____

_____

_____

My thoughts for today:

_____

_____

_____

_____

_____

April 11th

Thought of the Day

No one knows how much time we have on this earth. I think Muhammad Ali said it well: "Don't count the days, make the days count." There's no day like today to make a difference. Go get it!

My prayer for today is:

_____

_____

_____

What I will do today to exercise power in my life:

_____

_____

_____

_____

My thoughts for today:

_____

_____

_____

_____

April 12th

Thought of the Day

Tiger Woods won the 2019 Masters Golf Tournament. It's the perfect triumphant story of redemption. From being on top of the sports world to affairs, arrests, divorce, tons of medical problems, back to subpar golf, "experts" saying he was done, and another Masters win is phenomenal. You may have seen the picture of a guy standing by the golf course heckling Tiger wearing a T-shirt with Tiger's mugshot on it. Tiger never acknowledged it, Instead, he kept walking and ultimately won in grand fashion. Some people will forever highlight your past. But pull a "Tiger" and just keep walking because if God restored and refocused you, you'll see them again when you reach the winner's circle.

My prayer for today is:

_____

_____

_____

What I will do today to exercise power in my life:

_____

_____

_____

_____

My thoughts for today:

_____

_____

_____

_____

_____

April 13th

Thought of the Day

When I run a race, I can't help but look at people around me. There are the professionals who truly come to win the race. That's not my goal. However, I must admit that I am a little competitive. I often see people 20, 30, and even 40 years my senior out there. I tell myself that I can't let them beat me. But you know what, some of them do! Some of them have been running 50 years! They have the discipline, the stamina, and the endurance. I can't be mad at them. They put in the work. I actually smile when they cross the finish line. I'm happy for them, and I know I'll keep working to pass them. Most of all, I can't wait to leave youngsters in my dust in my later years. Do the work to reap the reward.

My prayer for today is:

_____

_____

_____

What I will do today to exercise power in my life:

_____

_____

_____

_____

My thoughts for today:

_____

_____

_____

_____

_____

April 14th

Thought of the Day

Your current situation is just right for God to show you, the enemy, and especially those who think they've got you cornered that He specializes in favoring those who are faithful to Him. Friend, keep pressing because God is working! Now, go have a blessed day!

My prayer for today is:

_____

_____

_____

What I will do today to exercise power in my life:

_____

_____

_____

_____

My thoughts for today:

_____

_____

_____

_____

_____

April 15th

Thought of the Day

I think you can find sermons everywhere. I found this sermon in a rap song , Nicki Minaj said *Everybody Dies But Not Everybody Lives*, Being born and dying are facts of life. Both of these things are out of our control. However, what we do between those two life events is up to us. We can choose to merely exist or we can live. When we live, we are intentional about making a difference. We can make a decision to optimize this thing called life. When this life is over, will your obituary show that you existed or that you lived? Go live your best life!

My prayer for today is:

_____

_____

_____

What I will do today to exercise power in my life:

_____

_____

_____

_____

My thoughts for today:

_____

_____

_____

_____

_____

April 16th

Thought of the Day

Very few people would watch their home burn and not call for firefighters who have the expertise and power to help. Very few of us would be very sick and not go to the doctor who has the expertise and power to help. God places people in our path to help and He keeps His ears open to our cries. He's omniscient—He knows all things. He's omnipresent—He's everywhere at the same time. And He's omnipotent—He's all-powerful. I think it's safe to say He's got the power and expertise to do ANYTHING but fail.

My prayer for today is:

_____

_____

_____

What I will do today to exercise power in my life:

_____

_____

_____

_____

My thoughts for today:

_____

_____

_____

_____

April 17th

Thought of the Day

The goodness and grace of God are so great that with every challenge God allows, it comes with a "God guarantee" that He's got your back no matter how it looks or feels. In other words, our Master will ensure you'll make it no matter what!

My prayer for today is:

_____

_____

_____

What I will do today to exercise power in my life:

_____

_____

_____

_____

My thoughts for today:

_____

_____

_____

_____

_____

April 18th

Thought of the Day

Simple word for you today, my friend. God is faithful! Therefore, there's no need for you to fail, to fall, to fret, or to let frustration rule your thoughts, emotions, or decisions. Trust God. Stand still and watch Him step right in and move on your behalf in His own timing and in His own way.

My prayer for today is:

_____

_____

_____

What I will do today to exercise power in my life:

_____

_____

_____

_____

My thoughts for today:

_____

_____

_____

_____

_____

April 19th

Thought of the Day

Understand that when it comes to life's paths, what's comfortable and convenient is not always what's productive and prosperous. Very often it's the challenges that create the open doors and opportunities that you've been praying and waiting for.

My prayer for today is:

_____

_____

_____

What I will do today to exercise power in my life:

_____

_____

_____

_____

My thoughts for today:

_____

_____

_____

_____

_____

April 20th

Thought of the Day

Have you ever seen the Farmers Insurance commercials that end with the line "We know a thing or two because we've seen a thing or two"? Well, God sends us the same message with a slight modification, "I know it all because I've seen it all." That's encouraging to the believer because there is not one thing our God doesn't see. Therefore, He not only sees our issues, He sees us through our issues. He also sees to it that we have what we need not only to make it but to be successful. Celebrate that God sees all, knows all, and does what it takes to take care of His own.

My prayer for today is:

_____

_____

_____

What I will do today to exercise power in my life:

_____

_____

_____

_____

My thoughts for today:

_____

_____

_____

_____

_____

April 21st

Thought of the Day

Too often we try to rationalize God instead of simply relying on Him through our faith. Keep in mind that the capacity of our little brains can't even begin to comprehend all God that directs and does. That's why our little hearts must have a big faith to trust and believe that God loves us and will continually lead us to our blessed places and lift us from our low places.

My prayer for today is:

_____

_____

_____

What I will do today to exercise power in my life:

_____

_____

_____

My thoughts for today:

_____

_____

_____

_____

_____

April 22nd

Thought of the Day

Never apologize to others for what God is doing in your life. The fact is, God didn't ask other people for their opinions before He blessed you. Therefore, you need not concern yourself with their opinions after He blesses you. Humbly receive what heaven releases and keep it moving!

My prayer for today is:

_____

_____

_____

What I will do today to exercise power in my life:

_____

_____

_____

_____

My thoughts for today:

_____

_____

_____

_____

_____

April 23rd

Thought of the Day

Little distractions can bring big destruction. Know that the enemy doesn't have to kill you to keep you from all that God has for you. Often it's the enemy's design to get you off course, even if just for a moment, so you'll miss opportunities and open doors. Keep your focus and keep the favor upon your life.

My prayer for today is:

_____

_____

_____

What I will do today to exercise power in my life:

_____

_____

_____

_____

My thoughts for today:

_____

_____

_____

_____

_____

April 24th

Thought of the Day

What is meant by the phrase "slept like a baby"? Babies sleep well when their needs have been met. They rest peacefully because they have no worries. Parents know that, because they are watching them sleep. They are watching their little chests rise and fall. They are making sure that all is well with their child. The fact that God never sleeps or even gets sleepy is a sufficient, comforting reason why His children should sleep like babies. He's always watching and at work on our behalf. The question is, are you doing the best you can and then turning the rest over to Him? My prayer is that you'll sleep like a baby.

My prayer for today is:

_____

_____

_____

What I will do today to exercise power in my life:

_____

_____

_____

_____

My thoughts for today:

_____

_____

_____

_____

April 25th

Thought of the Day

Don't worry when there are those who do their best to crucify your character. God has a successful history of resurrecting. For a Christian, the cross doesn't kill your spirit—it fills your spirit. Be revived with newfound focus and determination. Like the commercial I just saw, "the rival that's looking to take you down just takes your game higher." Rise from it!

My prayer for today is:

_____

_____

_____

What I will do today to exercise power in my life:

_____

_____

_____

_____

My thoughts for today:

_____

_____

_____

_____

_____

April 26th

Thought of the Day

Don't trip when someone says you're turning your back on them because you choose not to accept the invitation to their pity parties or the role they offer you in their daily dramas. You have something better to do with your time. If they are willing to walk *with* you toward something positive, they won't be looking at your back. You're going on a journey. Why would you weigh yourself down with someone else's baggage? Being a friend allows you to counsel someone on how to lighten a load. It doesn't mean getting weighed down by their load. There is a weight limit that must be observed for you to fly. Fly high today!

My prayer for today is:

_____

_____

_____

What I will do today to exercise power in my life:

_____

_____

_____

_____

My thoughts for today:

_____

_____

_____

_____

April 27th

Thought of the Day

Years ago, I had helped to get gospel aerobics started at my church. When some of the ladies who attended started to see results, they went into fitness mode and wanted to run a half marathon. They asked me to do it with them. My philosophy back then was that I only ran if something was chasing me. Nonetheless, I agreed to do it because we were on this fitness journey together. I trained so poorly, mostly because I didn't understand what proper training entailed. Another lady had also trained poorly. We showed up at the race. I remember us telling each other that we'd likely get separated during the race but no matter what, just finish. I remember being at the start line listening to Bishop Morton singing *Let it Rain* through my ear buds. We did both finish. A mere few months later, she passed away due to metastatic breast cancer. We were unaware of the diagnosis when we ran that race. I shortly signed up for another race to run in her memory. She wasn't overweight or obese, but for women who are, there is a higher risk for certain cancers. That's true for men as well. Run, walk, or whatever you can do for your life. I'd rather run for my life than to have others run in memory of my life. Get on the road to wellness and watch the blessings rain on your life. You have the power!

My prayer for today is:

_____

_____

_____

What I will do today to exercise power in my life:

_____

_____

_____

_____

My thoughts for today:

_____

_____

_____

_____

_____

April 28th

Thought of the Day

It seems to me Instagram takes a snapshot of who people are in that instant, that moment. Does it tell you who that person is for life? I'm not knocking Instagram. There are people promoting awareness and speaking positivity there. Take it in moderation, though. If you spend too much time watching others' lives, are you fully living yours? Social media is meant to influence. Have you noticed that people who are living their best lives have lots of followers but they don't follow many people themselves? They are hustling to build their brands. Don't learn your lessons from what they post. Learn from the habits they practice the most. Be the influencer, not the influenced.

My prayer for today is:

_____

_____

_____

What I will do today to exercise power in my life:

_____

_____

_____

_____

My thoughts for today:

_____

_____

_____

_____

_____

April 29th

Thought of the Day

Sometimes I don't know that it's getting older that we fear so much. Sometimes it's the stark reality of what we have yet to accomplish or the enormity of what we want to accomplish that freezes us in place. There is no way to move forward without taking a step. Take it one step at a time. In baseball, you score by crossing home plate. It doesn't mean you have to hit a home run every time. It's okay to start by just getting to first base. Batter up!

My prayer for today is:

_____

_____

_____

What I will do today to exercise power in my life:

_____

_____

_____

My thoughts for today:

_____

_____

_____

_____

_____

April 30th

Thought of the Day

Have you used a car service like Uber? You connect with a driver through an app. A person you don't know shows up who you believe will take you where you want to go. If you can trust this unknown person, how about truly exercising your faith in God? He knows where you want to go. Faith allows you to thank God for answering your prayers before it's confirmed that the prayers have been answered. Faith just knows that God has already done what you've asked Him to do. Be on your way by faith!

My prayer for today is:

_____

_____

_____

What I will do today to exercise power in my life:

_____

_____

_____

_____

My thoughts for today:

_____

_____

_____

_____

_____

May

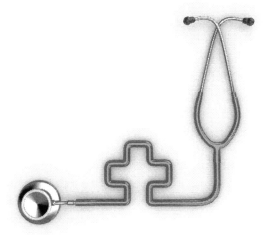

May
Mother, May I?

Medicine

Another crowded day at church is Mother's Day. Moms like showing off their babies even if the babies are 50 years old. Even those who have lost their mothers show up in reverence to others who have filled that role. The day pays respect to those who serve in the matriarch role along with those who are connected by blood or other close relationships. Arguably, there is nothing more powerful than a praying mother. It's not uncommon to see that big, tough defensive tackle on the NFL saying "hi" to his mother when the camera pans his way. We learn so much from our mother figures. Matriarchs are often the gateway to health for families.

Unfortunately, these wonderful women often neglect their own health due to their focus on caring for others. We commonly emulate their best traits. Likewise, we also pick up some of their bad habits and even pass them on. Sometimes, we respect our mothers so much, we don't want to question why they do or have done some of the things they have done.

In my own experience, I remember the women in my family questioning why I wanted to lay my newborn on his back to sleep. I heard, "You were laid on your stomach and you're here!" What did I know? I was just a doctor. My maternal grandmother died at 107 years of age. I still laugh when I think about how she told me, as I started to change my diet, that I started eating funny after I moved to Washington, D.C. I moved to D.C. from my home of Alabama. I traded my fried pork chops for grilled fish. My maternal grandfather raised pigs for income when I was growing up. Obviously, I am not knocking pork. It served my family well. I cannot deny that well-seasoned fried porkchops are tasty—at least to a lot of us from the South. However, neither can I deny the strokes that have occurred in every generation of my family.

There are many reasons our families have eaten the way they have. We can't ignore other pieces of the equation though. Many times our elders were more physically active in their daily vocations in comparison to the younger generations within the family. I love the big southern family meals we have shared. Those are great memories for sure. I even think there are still times for those types of celebrations. They should be the exceptions and not the rule. That's part of our history, but that doesn't mean we cannot or should not write new chapters. The Bible does say to honor your father and your mother. Preacher, what if we lived healthier lives so we could be around to honor them longer?

Ministry

At its core, honoring our mothers and fathers implies a few things. It means having and showing them the utmost respect. It means when life shifts the balance, children tend to and care for their parents just as their parents cared for them for so many years. It means valuing their sacrifices and the lessons they taught. And, yes, it also means lifting and illuminating their legacy for years and generations to come.

You spoke of Grandmother. She was something else, wasn't she? I mean, this is a lady who was hospitalized three times her whole life. Two of those times were within the last 2 years of her life. The other time was when she had her gall bladder removed when she was *younger*—in her 90s. God blessed her with great health. I remember one day our mother and her sister (whom we affectionately called *Sis*) were giving Grandmother the riot act about eating better. "What did they do that for?!" Grandmother responded, "I'm near 100 and have only been in the hospital one time in my life. And I've eaten everything and anything I want. Ya'll are the ones that stay sick!" She shut it down!

God graced Grandmother with longevity. However, I do believe that you are correct when saying we must take an honest and accurate assessment of our lineage, our raising, family traditions, and heredity. From a spiritual standpoint, we can't be afraid to confront things that have transcended generations. For example, you mentioned strokes. Diabetes is another culprit in our family. Cancer and hypertension have also been mainstays in our family lines. However, we're not alone. Most likely this is the truth for most people reading this book.

We must make some decisions that may break from what we've always known if it means better health and longevity. It doesn't mean our forefathers were wrong. It just means that God gives us wisdom, knowledge, and even technology that can help us live healthier lives. Not only that, but God has also given us spiritual power through His Son Jesus where we cannot only face some of these generational strongholds but defeat them. If God is for us, who can be against us?

May

Our hope for you this month is that you appreciate the role your family history has played in your life. It may emphasize habits you should keep or point out new traditions you want to start.

Plan to keep faith and wellness in the family. What are your goals for this month?

1.

2.

3.

May 1st

Thought of the Day

Sometimes we strive so hard to get to that perfect picture of who we want to be that we don't appreciate how the puzzle pieces are coming together to create that picture. As the saying goes, don't let perfect be the enemy of good. We are works in progress. Celebrate each milestone along the way.

My prayer for today is:

_____

_____

_____

What I would like to pass on:

_____

_____

_____

_____

My thoughts for today:

_____

_____

_____

_____

May 2nd

Thought of the Day

I appreciate every elevation to which God has taken me. Even though I may be going on to something bigger and better, it is not unusual for it to also come with bigger challenges. I wouldn't take anything for my journey, but I have learned to pray for strength for the journey. My friends, be ready to go places but don't forget to pack your prayer and your faith.

My prayer for today is:

_____

_____

_____

What I would like to pass on:

_____

_____

_____

_____

My thoughts for today:

_____

_____

_____

_____

_____

May 3ʳᵈ

Thought of the Day

Maya Angelou once said, "I've learned that people will forget what you said, people will forget what you did, but people will never forget how you made them feel." Sometimes people may not like you, but they can't deny that you always treated them fairly. When we put this into practice, it comes down to treating others the way you want to be treated. Before you treat someone out of your emotions, bring back that timeless question, "What would Jesus do?"

My prayer for today is:

_____

_____

_____

What I would like to pass on:

_____

_____

_____

_____

My thoughts for today:

_____

_____

_____

_____

_____

May 4th

Thought of the Day

One of the things I've learned through my work is that you can have the best intentions when you're trying to give people the things that you think they need. It hurts when they don't seem to appreciate your efforts. Sometimes, it's not that they aren't grateful but it just may be that what you're giving is not what they need the most. It's like giving a person food to cook but their electricity has been disconnected. Likewise, we don't always tell people what we need from them. The best exchanges in life are fulfilling for both the giver and the receiver. If you listen to what people need, you won't be giving them a handout, you'll be giving them a hand.

My prayer for today is:

_____

_____

_____

What I would like to pass on:

_____

_____

_____

_____

My thoughts for today:

_____

_____

_____

_____

_____

May 5th

Thought of the Day

I love the spiritual that says, "May the work I've done speak for me. May the life I've lived, speak for me. Lord, when I'm resting in my grave, I know there's nothing that can be said. May the work I've done speak for me." My prayer is that you walk in your purpose and that it speaks volumes of who you are. Be blessed!

My prayer for today is:

_____

_____

_____

What I would like to pass on:

_____

_____

_____

_____

My thoughts for today:

_____

_____

_____

_____

_____

May 6th

Thought of the Day

Steve Prefontaine said, "To give anything less than your best, is to sacrifice the gift." You can quietly thank God for the gift that He's given you. However, if you proudly and openly share your gift to the best of your ability, you not only honor Him many times over but it's likely that many others are blessed in the process. No one has ever been recognized as gifted if they haven't shared their gift. Don't discount the power of your gift.

My prayer for today is:

_____

_____

_____

What I would like to pass on:

_____

_____

_____

_____

My thoughts for today:

_____

_____

_____

_____

May 7th

Thought of the Day

The spirit with which you do something matters. A positive attitude tramples dread. I have started doing some interactive spin classes. On the screen, I follow the instructor and can see how I'm doing as well. I don't mind that I'm dripping in sweat because I enjoy the positive spirit of the instructors. Not only does your spirit matter but it influences others. Let your spirit bless others today. You could really help them over a hard time.

My prayer for today is:

_____

_____

_____

What I would like to pass on:

_____

_____

_____

_____

My thoughts for today:

_____

_____

_____

_____

_____

May 8th

Thought of the Day

There is a bakery café in my hometown that makes the best homemade cakes. I swear, caramel cake is my kryptonite. It calls my name, and my stomach wants to bypass my brain and answer every single time! My caramel-loving stomach tries hard to convince me that I need a slice or two—maybe three. I do treat myself to a slice from time to time when I go home. But do you know what stops me from eating half of the cake? I don't bring it home with me! Willpower is about making the right choices. Sometimes the right choice is to remove the temptation altogether. Be your best superman or superwoman. Don't let your kryptonite cripple you!

My prayer for today is:

_____

_____

_____

What I would like to pass on:

_____

_____

_____

_____

My thoughts for today:

_____

_____

_____

_____

May 9th

Thought of the Day

We always want to see our children do better than we did. Often we apply that to making sure they have more than we had. I think we've all seen enough examples that having more material things does not make the next generation better. We need to make sure they have more of the building blocks for the best life. Are we passing on good work ethics, good self-esteem habits, and healthy habits? These are the things that will last when material things are gone.

My prayer for today is:

_____

_____

_____

What I would like to pass on:

_____

_____

_____

_____

My thoughts for today:

_____

_____

_____

_____

_____

May 10ᵗʰ

Thought of the Day

Some of you can remember the days when, as kids, we spent hours playing outside. We walked for hours in the mall. Those things seemed like normal life. A positive side effect was that we were moving. Today, video games keep too many of us tied to a couch or chair. We shop online.Excessive sitting has now even been likened to smoking in terms of the potential impact on your health   We call these things technological advances, but they are not advancing our health, at least not when we use them in excess. Find a balance with technology. They should augment your life—not stop you from living it. Get moving!

My prayer for today is:

_____

_____

_____

What I would like to pass on:

_____

_____

_____

_____

My thoughts for today:

_____

_____

_____

_____

May 11th

Thought of the Day

Years ago, we heard our mother screaming from the back of the house. We rushed to see what was wrong. She was trying on spring and summer clothes she had stored in suitcases over the winter. She declared that the suitcases had shrunken her clothes. If you have devious suitcases like the ones she had, diet and exercise helps to negate their power.

My prayer for today is:

_____

_____

_____

What I would like to pass on:

_____

_____

_____

_____

My thoughts for today:

_____

_____

_____

_____

_____

May 12th

Thought of the Day

It's incumbent on all of us to make sure that we're aligned with God, His Word, and His Spirit. It's so vital because if we're not aligned with God, then those who align with us will be misaligned in so many areas of their life. Don't you be responsible for another person's "crooked places."

My prayer for today is:

_____

_____

_____

What I would like to pass on:

_____

_____

_____

_____

My thoughts for today:

_____

_____

_____

_____

May 13th

Thought of the Day

The best part of your day is the fact that you're still here to enjoy it! Don't complain today. Celebrate life above all else. Then you and God can handle whatever life throws your way.

My prayer for today is:

_____

_____

_____

What I would like to pass on:

_____

_____

_____

_____

My thoughts for today:

_____

_____

_____

_____

_____

May 14th

Thought of the Day

It's YOUR faith! That means you're not dependent on what others think or believe. It's a matter of what YOUR heart says. It is a matter of what YOUR heart believes. It's a matter of YOUR mind being able to conceive YOURSELF as better, as blessed, as healed, as helped, as independent, as successful, as whatever. What's the verdict about YOUR life? Consult YOUR heart, YOUR mind, YOUR faith, and YOUR God for the answers.

My prayer for today is:

_____

_____

_____

What I would like to pass on:

_____

_____

_____

_____

My thoughts for today:

_____

_____

_____

_____

_____

May 15th

Thought of the Day

Focus! People are going to think what they think. They're also going to do what they do! But you and God control your narrative. Write your story through the lens of your faith and focus without looking in any direction but forward and upward.

My prayer for today is:

_____

_____

_____

What I would like to pass on:

_____

_____

_____

_____

My thoughts for today:

_____

_____

_____

_____

May 16th

Thought of the Day

Three words to make you rejoice regarding what you need from God, what you're believing God to do, and the desires of your heart: IT'S ALREADY DONE! Your faithfulness to God is being met by His faithfulness to you.

My prayer for today is:

_____

_____

_____

What I would like to pass on:

_____

_____

_____

_____

My thoughts for today:

_____

_____

_____

_____

_____

May 17th

Thought of the Day

Do things in such a way that others are blessed and God is glorified. Our Father will ensure that you are acknowledged, blessed, elevated, exalted, promoted, and shown favor at the right time, at the right place, by the right people, and in front of the right people. It is so!

My prayer for today is:

_____

_____

_____

What I would like to pass on:

_____

_____

_____

My thoughts for today:

_____

_____

_____

_____

May 18th

Thought of the Day

Why should we be surprised if others don't believe in us when we don't believe in ourselves? If we want others to give us a chance, we must show that we are worth it. If you need positive affirmations to start your day, put that sticky note on your mirror to serve as your mini pep talk. When you look at your mirror, you'll see positive words and the person who deserves them! If writing notes isn't your thing, you can just thank God for both your person and your purpose. Thank Him for loving you. To acknowledge that He loves you should affirm that you are worthy! Walk out that door today with your head held high!

My prayer for today is:

_____

_____

_____

What I would like to pass on:

_____

_____

_____

_____

My thoughts for today:

_____

_____

_____

_____

_____

May 19th

Thought of the Day

Few of us throw away our phones, tablets, or other devices because their batteries are drained, empty, or dead. We just recharge the batteries and reboot the devices so they can continue doing what they were created to do. That's your word, my friend. So you feel drained, empty, and maybe even emotionally, mentally, and spiritually dead. Pause with the pity party! Go to God. Be transparent about your situations and how you're feeling. Allow God to recharge you and reboot you. Then you go back to doing great things and glorifying God. After all, that's what you were created to do!

My prayer for today is:

_____

_____

_____

What I would like to pass on:

_____

_____

_____

_____

My thoughts for today:

_____

_____

_____

_____

_____

May 20th

Thought of the Day

One who really understands how fragile, short, and unpredictable life is has no reservations and needs no motivation in appreciating another day that the Lord has given to him or her. This person also is very intentional about not wasting one second of this precious day on things that don't matter. Make it a productive day!

My prayer for today is:

_____

_____

_____

What I would like to pass on:

_____

_____

_____

_____

My thoughts for today:

_____

_____

_____

_____

_____

May 21st

Thought of the Day

I have wonderful neighbors who are so genuine in spirit. They watch my house when I'm away. They've been a blessing to my son. They help me troubleshoot when things aren't working right at my house. They are truly godly people. They've recently become new parents. I think sleep deprivation sometimes makes them question if they're good parents. Here's what I know. They have been genuinely nurturing in every aspect of their lives. God was allowing them to practice the very foundations of good parenting even before their beautiful baby was in her womb. The same God who blessed them to conceive, is the same God who will continue with them in this parenting journey. They are great parents because they have learned from their Father. My hope for you is that others will see in you what you've learned from the Father. Be blessed.

My prayer for today is:

_____

_____

_____

What I would like to pass on:

_____

_____

_____

_____

My thoughts for today:

_____

_____

_____

_____

May 22nd

Thought of the Day

Growing up, my grandmother would cook the best turnip greens imaginable! Part or the reason they were so good is because she'd put a ham hock or a piece of "fat back" into the pot with the greens to provide seasoning. (My sister would vote for a smoked turkey wing.) Anyway, what she added provided flavor to the pot. Sometimes God strategically places us with people and in situations for one reason: to "season the pot." He desires us to "flavor" the atmosphere and the people with whom we come into contact with the joy, peace, happiness, faith, love, and power of Christ. After all, Jesus said we are the "salt of the earth." If that be the case, friend, get salty for the Savior!

My prayer for today is:

_____

_____

_____

What I would like to pass on:

_____

_____

_____

_____

My thoughts for today:

_____

_____

_____

_____

_____

May 23rd

Thought of the Day

Don't use your family as excuses. Specifically, don't use your family history as a reason to not try. High blood pressure may run in your family. There may be a pattern of mental health issues in your family. Maybe you were diagnosed with Type I diabetes as a child. Just because you were born with a genetic predisposition for certain conditions does not give you a pass from trying to live your best life. As a matter of fact, if your behavior exacerbates the situation, you'll be living your worst life. Family history play a significant role in how you start, but it doesn't dictate how you end. Get going on changing your family story!

My prayer for today is:

_____

_____

_____

What I would like to pass on:

_____

_____

_____

_____

My thoughts for today:

_____

_____

_____

_____

_____

May 24th

Thought of the Day

At my company and many others, we do succession planning. That is basically creating a plan on who will occupy your seat if you were to leave the firm. It makes you stay grounded in knowing that nothing is promised and nothing lasts forever. It also makes you think about the legacy you want to leave and what steps you have taken to create a lasting legacy. It means shaping others and supporting them to be ready to take your spot. Here's the thing, if you are really striving to do a great work that will serve others, you should want that good work to live past you. It's bigger than you or at least it should be. Look for those successors who share your vision and will have the energy and commitment to take that forward. It doesn't mean they won't shape things their way, but the core of what you stand for should remain. I believe you have successors not only in the workplace but in life. What is the legacy you want to live on? Have you lived by example for your children, grandchildren, and others so that what sprouts from that seed continues to grow? Be well in body, mind, and spirit. I believe that is something that we want to pass on and have live on in all that we touch.

My prayer for today is:

_____

_____

_____

What I would like to pass on:

_____

_____

_____

_____

My thoughts for today:

_____

_____

_____

_____

_____

May 25th

Thought of the Day

Often it isn't that God doesn't desire to move in your situation. It's that God is waiting for you to move out of the way and for you to take your agenda, plans, and thinking with you. Sometimes we can't resist trying things our way. When my brother and I were kids, we went to a carnival and entered this house that contained a maze constructed of glass walls. We thought it would be easy to get out. It looked clear. What could be hard about that? It wasn't long before we realized that it wasn't easy at all. We kept running into glass walls. We started to panic. We realized if we listened to the voices of people coming in, we could find our way out. (Okay, so we went back out the front instead of making it to the back.) The point is that sometimes we try to go our own way in life, but if we listen to God's voice, we can make it through this big maze we call life.

My prayer for today is:

_____

_____

_____

What I would like to pass on:

_____

_____

_____

_____

My thoughts for today:

_____

_____

_____

_____

_____

May 26th

Thought of the Day

The moment that you can honestly look in the mirror with determination and say "I'm better than this" is the moment you begin the journey to be better than what you see. Self-improvement begins with self-assessment. It continues with self-motivation and self-accountability. Keep on your journey!

My prayer for today is:

_____

_____

_____

What I would like to pass on:

_____

_____

_____

_____

My thoughts for today:

_____

_____

_____

_____

_____

May 27th

Thought of the Day

Facing today is not nearly as hard as you think when you remember who it was that kept you, provided for you, and protected you yesterday. Be thankful that we serve an immutable God. That is, He's the same God all the time. Celebrate that He is your covering. You can walk confidently even though there may be the threat of storms.

My prayer for today is:

_____

_____

_____

What I would like to pass on:

_____

_____

_____

_____

My thoughts for today:

_____

_____

_____

_____

_____

May 28th

Thought of the Day

The excitement and expectation that you have about something creates the drive and dedication you'll have to stay strong, focused, and patient and see your vision through. Nobody else can live out your dream. It's on you this blessed day.

My prayer for today is:

_____

_____

_____

What I would like to pass on:

_____

_____

_____

_____

My thoughts for today:

_____

_____

_____

_____

_____

May 29th

Thought of the Day

Trusting God equates to getting into the passenger seat of a car, relaxing, and enjoying the ride while someone else has full control of the vehicle and ultimately of your welfare and your life. Trusting God simply says, "Lord, my life is in your hands. I'm going to relax and ride because I know you're in control of where I'm going, how I'm getting there, and my welfare during the journey." Give God full control!

My prayer for today is:

_____

_____

_____

What I would like to pass on:

_____

_____

_____

_____

My thoughts for today:

_____

_____

_____

_____

_____

May 30th

Thought of the Day

I hope you are excited about transitioning to a healthy lifestyle! Don't skip over the fact that "lifestyle" does mean a new way of living forever. In your excitement, don't start so aggressively that it's something you can't sustain. You've heard in relationships, the things you do to win someone over are the same things you need to keep doing to keep them. It's the same way with the healthy lifestyle you're trying to achieve. I often liken a healthy lifestyle to the Christian journey. It's day by day and sometimes tough, but it's worth it. Push yourself, but choose a path that you can continue to follow for the long run.

My prayer for today is:

_____

_____

_____

What I would like to pass on:

_____

_____

_____

_____

My thoughts for today:

_____

_____

_____

_____

_____

May 31st

Thought of the Day

I'll never forget when I was young, my sister, our cousin, our boxer (dog) Benji, and I went with my dad to pick up his check. He worked for over 30 years at a plant that bordered the Tennessee River. When he got his check, we went to the plant's park. My dad grabbed Benji and hurled him into the river! We were beside ourselves screaming "Daaaadddy! He'll drown." Daddy said, "He can swim. He's just never had to. He'll be fine." Lo and behold, Benji calmly swam back to shore—and then jumped in a few more times. Your word is simple, friend! Sometimes God allows things in our lives to bring out of us the ability and potential that we've never tapped into before. No matter the issue, "don't drown!" Be like Benji and work out what's in you! It's sink or swim time! Now SWIM, SURVIVE, and SUCCEED!

My prayer for today is:

_____

_____

_____

What I would like to pass on:

_____

_____

_____

My thoughts for today:

_____

_____

_____

_____

June

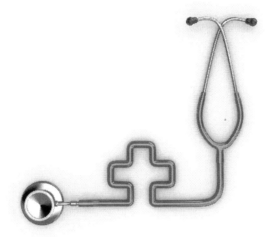

June
Graduation

Medicine

I had envisioned my medical school graduation so many times. I started dreaming of it when I was a child. I could see myself practically dancing across the stage with a big smile on my face. By the time that day actually came, there were over 190 others in the line ahead of me. While medical school was rewarding, it was also challenging on so many levels. It tested my intellect, emotional stability, and even physical stamina. I kept thinking that degree had better actually be within the covers of that leather folder or I'd stage a bitter protest right there!

The image I had of practically floating across the stage was based on my passively receiving the honor. The reality, after countless hours in the library and the hospital, was that I actively earned every single letter on that degree. It was a confirmation that I was committed to serving others through medicine. It was a reminder of all I sacrificed for the purpose of being a servant. I crossed the finish line but could not deny there was some wear and tear on my body and soul for the journey. It's amazing how the songs we've repeatedly heard come back to us. Frankly, sometimes we even resented the fact that our parents made us listen to those verses in what seemed like eternal repeat mode. Countless times in my house growing up, I heard the lyrics, "Oh, Jesus, you don't have to move my mountain. Just give me the strength to climb." It sometimes pained me then, but I can't tell you how many times in medical school it comforted and fortified my spirit.

The point of matriculation through any schooling is to learn and to leave better than you came. The real success in education is applying what you've learned in life. When it comes to health, there is some knowledge that you actually gather in school whether in a biology, anatomy, or physiology class.

We also learn a lot outside of the classroom when we see loved ones suffer or die from preventable conditions related to things like obesity. We see equations for disaster lived out in the real world daily. However, we know how to solve the problem. Why don't we? Is it because it's hard? The very nature of problem solving is to overcome the challenges. It is often said, when you know better, you do better. That's not always the case when it comes to living a healthier lifestyle. Children grow up in a lifestyle. We as adults know better. First Corinthians 13:11 (NLT) says, "When I was a child, I spoke as a child, I understood as a child, I thought as a child; but when I became a man, I put away childish things." Preacher, does that only apply to spiritual things?

Ministry

No, it doesn't only apply to spiritual things. However, I believe the whole idea of knowing better and doing better has spirituality as its root. It's about maturity and mindset. In both of these cases, God is ultimately the One who matures us and gives us the right mindset to ensure we do what's necessary to live our best life. Our Father uses many things to help us grow daily and to shape our thinking, our goals, our determination, and our discipline. Life experiences—either our own or the challenges of those we love—have a way of affecting us.

For example, our maternal grandfather, affectionately known as Papa, died in 1985 after a long, sad, and serious bout with lung cancer. Growing up, I can remember Papa as a very heavy smoker who puffed multiple packs of cigarettes per day. While I was just 12 years old when he died, I still remember vividly the toll that cancer took on him. I visited him at the hospital with Dad one day. Papa asked me to help him go to the bathroom. The flimsy hospital gown he wore came open in the back. I was surprised and startled by what I saw. Papa was emaciated—skin and bones. Lung cancer had reduced him to nothing. That day I declared that I'd never, ever smoke anything. To this day, as of this writing, I'm 47 years old, I have kept my vow.

Because of that one visual, and because cancer took away one of my childhood heroes, I detested cigarettes then and still do now. Our family can attest to the fact that during childhood, the first thing I'd do in any room I walked into was dump ashtrays. I literally couldn't eat if I saw dirty ashtrays. To even see cigarette butts on the ground today bothers me. And it all stems back to 1985. That image of Papa and his ultimate death shaped me forever and caused me to decide to never pollute my body with smoking materials of any kind.

Perhaps someone reading has had a similar experience with a loved one and serious medical conditions. Maybe you're currently the caretaker of a loved one with a preventable medical condition. Maybe you've vowed never to go down the same path that led to physical and emotional pain your loved one and the entire family are experiencing. If so, ask God to give you the determination and discipline to do what's necessary to change that narrative so it doesn't affect your life. Jesus said in John 14 that whatever we ask in His name, He'll do. So go ahead and ask for that help and determination. Then trust God to give you the wherewithal to make healthy choices and lifestyle changes.

June

Our hope for you is that you take things to the next level in your life. What are your goals for this month?

1.

2.

3.

June 1ˢᵗ

Thought of the Day

Have you ever been on a weight-loss journey and been doing well? All of a sudden, you hit the dreaded plateau. What you have been doing doesn't seem to work anymore. You try tweaks to your regimen, and that doesn't seem to work either. It makes you question if you should just give up. Geologically, a plateau is a high plain. It sits significantly above the surrounding area. In other words, it's not the peak but it's not the valley. Don't let your plateau make you forget that you have made a climb. You may not be where you want to be, but you're not where you were. Resolve that you will continue to focus on the peak ahead and not return to the valley.

My prayer for today is:

_____

_____

_____

What I will do today to go to the next level in my life:

_____

_____

_____

_____

My thoughts for today:

_____

_____

_____

_____

_____

June 2nd

Thought of the Day

Michelle Obama had a great saying, "When they go low, we go high." Some thought this statement indicated a passive stance. I disagree. This quote says to me that not only should we resist the urge to stoop to the level of someone aiming to bring us down but we should use their bluster as a tailwind to help us soar even higher. Fly high, my friends!

My prayer for today is:

_____

_____

_____

What I will do today to go to the next level in my life:

_____

_____

_____

_____

My thoughts for today:

_____

_____

_____

_____

_____

June 3rd

Thought of the Day

Broken people don't need a lecture about how they got broken. In fact, initially they don't need to be levied with a list of Scriptures either. Broken people immediately need love and lifting from people who know what brokenness looks like and feels like because they've just gotten put back together themselves. Your test and your testimony of how you made it through is often the tether that keeps a broken person from becoming scattered pieces never to be restored again. Be a difference-maker for someone else.

My prayer for today is:

_____

_____

_____

What I will do today to go to the next level in my life:

_____

_____

_____

_____

My thoughts for today:

_____

_____

_____

_____

_____

June 4th

Thought of the Day

There are so many good lines in the song *I Hope you Dance*, written by Tia and Mark Sanders. Some of my favorites include "I hope you never fear those mountains in the distance. Never settle for the path of least resistance. Living might mean taking chances, but they're worth taking. Loving might be a mistake, but it's worth making." It goes on to say, "Promise me that you'll give faith a fighting chance. And when you get the choice to sit it out or dance, dance." Life is worth living. You get the most out of it when you put your all in it. Friends, I truly hope you allow yourself to dance.

My prayer for today is:

_____

_____

_____

What I will do today to go to the next level in my life:

_____

_____

_____

_____

My thoughts for today:

_____

_____

_____

_____

_____

June 5th

Thought of the Day

We can't sit back and wait for good things to fall in our laps. God's goodness does not exempt us from doing our part to bring blessings to fruition. John F. Kennedy said, "Things do not happen. Things are made to happen." There is no day like today to make good things happen. Get to it!

My prayer for today is:

_____

_____

_____

What I will do today to go to the next level in my life:

_____

_____

_____

_____

My thoughts for today:

_____

_____

_____

_____

_____

June 6th

Thought of the Day

It is so easy to order food online. I've certainly been guilty. You can order a feast, and it shows up at your door. Lots of times that delivery comes in a really greasy bag or box. There are ways to help curb those habits. If you really need food from a certain restaurant, pick it up yourself. If you're struggling with the thought of going out to pick it up, you probably don't need it that badly. Stock your refrigerator and cabinets with healthy food so when a craving hit, you have good alternatives available. It takes away the argument that there was only junk food to eat. Finally, you can meal prep for the week. It takes some time on the weekends, but it saves time on the weekdays. It balances out. Stack the odds in your favor of winning your fight!

My prayer for today is:

_____

_____

_____

What I will do today to go to the next level in my life:

_____

_____

_____

_____

My thoughts for today:

_____

_____

_____

_____

_____

June 7th

Thought of the Day

Our dad has Type 2 diabetes despite his eating pretty well and staying active. He doesn't spend time on thinking his diagnosis is unfair. He uses it as motivation to keep himself active. He walks almost daily on a track. When it came to optimizing his health, attitude was the first thing he had to deal with. It could either propel him forward or weigh him down. I'm proud to say he continues to get around that track faster and faster.

My prayer for today is:

_____

_____

_____

What I will do today to go to the next level in my life:

_____

_____

_____

_____

My thoughts for today:

_____

_____

_____

_____

_____

June 8th

Thought of the Day

None of us have the ability to retrieve time. That's why it's so prudent that we honor and respect every precious second the good Lord gives us and demand that others do the same. It's on YOU if you dishonor and waste time. It's also on YOU if you continually allow others to disrespect your time. You and everything concerning you are too valuable for that!

My prayer for today is:

_____

_____

_____

What I will do today to go to the next level in my life:

_____

_____

_____

_____

My thoughts for today:

_____

_____

_____

_____

June 9th

Thought of the Day

The first year I applied to medical school, there was a glitch in the centralized system that was supposed to electronically deliver my application to the various medical schools in which I was interested. I was not hearing anything when others around me were receiving correspondence from their schools. I ended up getting a few interviews at schools that had already filled their classes. I was put on a wait list and didn't move up. I didn't even apply the next year because I was so devastated. I worked at a power company steam plant. When I decided to pursue my dream again, I found myself on the steps of Georgetown University School of Medicine. The university seal was on the floor of the lobby. Before I went into my interviews, I stood on that seal and declared I was home. Georgetown welcomed me, and I never looked back. Georgetown had not been on my list before then. I look back and, as funny as it sounds, I am so grateful that the other schools didn't work out. Georgetown opened so many doors for me. I am extremely proud of my alma mater. We've heard it before but I know the saying to be true, "delayed is not denied."

My prayer for today is:

_____

_____

_____

What I will do today to go to the next level in my life:

_____

_____

_____

_____

My thoughts for today:

_____

_____

_____

_____

_____

June 10th

Thought of the Day

Don't let others' reasons and excuses why you can't do something deter you. Instead, let those reasons and excuses be a part of the drive deep within you that causes you to EXPECT great things for your life. That drive should also push you to excel while you execute the plan you and God have devised that will lead you to achieving every hope and dream you have!

My prayer for today is:

_____

_____

_____

What I will do today to go to the next level in my life:

_____

_____

_____

_____

My thoughts for today:

_____

_____

_____

_____

_____

June 11th

Thought of the Day

Trusting God is saying and believing that something is or will be even while it's still just a hope and a dream. If you don't fully believe in yourself and in your God, then don't expect anyone else to embrace and celebrate your hopes and dreams and commit to helping you turn them into reality. YOUR heart sets the foundation for what's going to happen in your future.

My prayer for today is:

_____

_____

_____

What I will do today to go to the next level in my life:

_____

_____

_____

_____

My thoughts for today:

_____

_____

_____

_____

_____

June 12th

Thought of the Day

Becoming a difference-maker most often doesn't occur at the moment a difference is needed to be made. It happens over time as a person develops meaningful relationships, an honorable reputation, and an unusual resolve to be impactful and to be insightful no matter the circumstance or the crowd. These foundations are critical to the overall mission of making any kind of difference in any situation.

My prayer for today is:

_____

_____

_____

What I will do today to go to the next level in my life:

_____

_____

_____

_____

My thoughts for today:

_____

_____

_____

_____

_____

June 13th

Thought of the Day

We've all seen how car dealerships start advertising "inventory sales" in the fall. They want to sell what they have on the lot to make room for their new cars. The cars on the lot still look good. The new cars may not look any different on the outside but they often have improvements like new technology and new safety features. Today is your day of inventory. Who or what is stifling, smothering, or hindering your growth or the blessings designed for your life? Maybe it's time get rid of some of your old stock to make room for the new and improved you.

My prayer for today is:

_____

_____

_____

What I will do today to go to the next level in my life:

_____

_____

_____

_____

My thoughts for today:

_____

_____

_____

_____

_____

June 14th

Thought of the Day

Actions and reactions born out of ignorance, impulse, and erratic emotions never yield fruitful results or resolve. Calm down. Let things play out. Consider all of the facts. At that point, you can ponder the proper response and plan of execution. Immediacy is not always in your best interest.

My prayer for today is:

_____

_____

_____

What I will do today to go to the next level in my life:

_____

_____

_____

_____

My thoughts for today:

_____

_____

_____

_____

_____

June 15th

Thought of the Day

These days you hear so many commercials and commentaries on someone "being elite." This term implies a person, be it anyone from an athlete to someone in so many different professions, is head and shoulders above everyone else. But what's often not said is to be elite, one must first "be at least." Be at least passionate about what you're doing. Be at least committed to work and grind to get better and excel. Be at least selfless in order to make others around you better. And be at least grateful to God for talents, gifts, open doors, and opportunities. Strive to BE ELITE. But first ask God to help you BE AT LEAST.

My prayer for today is:

_____

_____

_____

What I will do today to go to the next level in my life:

_____

_____

_____

_____

My thoughts for today:

_____

_____

_____

_____

_____

June 16th

Thought of the Day

Never let anyone make you feel bad for having "a moment" when life presents hurts, tears, frustration, and disappointment. It's natural. It's okay. The key is making sure the moment doesn't become a mindset and a road map for your future. With God's help, and in His timing, you'll get through that rough season. Then you've got to get up, move on, and keep living. There is too much ahead to allow moments to become permanent.

My prayer for today is:

_____

_____

_____

What I will do today to go to the next level in my life:

_____

_____

_____

_____

My thoughts for today:

_____

_____

_____

_____

_____

June 17th

Thought of the Day

How many times have we complained that there is just not enough time to get things done, as we objectively took inventory of where our time went, for instance, participating in social media or watching reality TV? Even crazier, how many times have we seen on social media that our favorite reality TV star has been exposed for not having as much as they proclaimed to have? Not only have we invested time in them, we have bought into their lie. Don't spend so much time watching fake "reality" that your real life passes you by. Turn off the TV, and turn on your potential!

My prayer for today is:

_____

_____

_____

What I will do today to go to the next level in my life:

_____

_____

_____

_____

My thoughts for today:

_____

_____

_____

_____

_____

June 18th

Thought of the Day

I watched the documentary *Amazing Grace* about a live gospel performance by the late Aretha Franklin. Something about that documentary gave me chills. There was no superstar air about her. There were no elaborate special effects. It is flat-out singing! She is hardly captured speaking at all. She seems to be singing straight to God, and we have the honor of bearing witness to that through this documentary. It was like she could see God and was singing her path to heaven. I will never be able to sing like Aretha, but I can utilize the talents that I have been blessed with to pave my road to heaven day to day. Are you paving your way?

My prayer for today is:

_____

_____

_____

What I will do today to go to the next level in my life:

_____

_____

_____

_____

My thoughts for today:

_____

_____

_____

_____

June 19th

Thought of the Day

I still have connections with a couple of my elementary school teachers (shout-out to Mrs. Newman and Mrs. Hayden). They still celebrate accomplishments in my life. That means a lot, and I'm thankful for their influence on my life. My late maternal aunt, Mildred Turner, was also one of my teachers. I still tell people at work when reviewing a document, my aunt would not be happy with me if I let this go out written this way. I have to recognize teachers here because they don't get paid enough for what they do. They have the huge responsibility of shaping the minds of tomorrow. I believe good teachers are called. They pay it forward. With every success we have that has stemmed from a seed they have planted, we should thank God for them. Teachers are great examples that it doesn't take a large salary to make a huge impact. Use your gifts and talents to make a difference. It's your turn to pay it forward.

My prayer for today is:

_____

_____

_____

What I will do today to go to the next level in my life:

_____

_____

_____

_____

My thoughts for today:

_____

_____

_____

_____

_____

June 20th

Thought of the Day

I don't mind my friends pushing me. At least that way I know they've got my back! As Proverbs 27:17 (NIV) says, "iron sharpens iron." I like having friends who are go-getters. They have both faith and fortitude. That means I am further motivated not to become complacent. Surround yourself by those who push you and who like to be pushed back! Go get it!

My prayer for today is:

_____

_____

_____

What I will do today to go to the next level in my life:

_____

_____

_____

_____

My thoughts for today:

_____

_____

_____

_____

June 21st

Thought of the Day

There is method in what we perceive as madness. The process that God intends for us does not change. Sometimes we can't understand His process. So really it's a matter of our attitude and perspective while going through the process. Either we'll walk in fear or walk in faith. Either we'll be positive or we'll panic. Either we'll worship while we walk it out or we'll worry. We are the ones who most often determine how pleasant or how painful our journey is going to be. The journey is going to happen. How will you equip yourself for it?

My prayer for today is:

_____

_____

_____

What I will do today to go to the next level in my life:

_____

_____

_____

_____

My thoughts for today:

_____

_____

_____

_____

_____

June 22nd

Thought of the Day

I still believe. Even though there are some terrible things going on in this world, I still believe there are more good people than there are bad. I still believe that I can make a difference in this world. I still believe that there are many who feel the same way I do. I even believe that if we all come together, the world will be a different place. I believe God will answer our prayers. I believe that I am worth fighting for. I believe I have to fight for my wellness in body, mind, and spirit. In those moments that my flesh surfaces doubt, God, please help my unbelief. Belief is a daily, active exercise and never a passive proposition. Believe today and every day!

My prayer for today is:

_____

_____

_____

What I will do today to go to the next level in my life:

_____

_____

_____

My thoughts for today:

_____

_____

_____

_____

June 23rd

Thought of the Day

There comes a time when one must speak better and greater things over his or her own life. That applies to all aspects of our lives—better health, better job, better relationships. To speak those things doesn't mean they'll happen automatically. However, speaking great things over your own life should adjust your attitude, mindset, and motivation to do everything within your might to ensure your hopes and dreams become reality. Do we mean it when we say that we can do all things through Christ? "Do" is a verb—an action. Speaking should spark you to action. Let's go!

My prayer for today is:

_____

_____

_____

What I will do today to go to the next level in my life:

_____

_____

_____

_____

My thoughts for today:

_____

_____

_____

_____

_____

June 24th

Thought of the Day

Make up your mind to exercise, and see what your friends say. Do you have a friend who will fall back on the argument that they are just big-boned so exercise won't help? Will you have one that says they don't want to mess up their hair? Do you have one who will say before you start you should go out for one last really big meal? Guys, will your friends start recalling when they were buff in the past like that means something for the present and the future? If you can stay determined and push past your friends' excuses for not joining you, congratulations! You have completed tough exercise number one. Now, onto your new lifestyle!

My prayer for today is:

_____

_____

_____

What I will do today to go to the next level in my life:

_____

_____

_____

_____

My thoughts for today:

_____

_____

_____

_____

_____

June 25th

Thought of the Day

The only thing you should quit trying to do is the very thing that God told you not to do. It might be hard to not go where you used to or to stay away from those bad habits you used to have. But, rest assured that if you are in His will, you are backed by His Word. Your hard work will pay off. That's because He will make sure that not only will everything work out, it will work better.

My prayer for today is:

_____

_____

_____

What I will do today to go to the next level in my life:

_____

_____

_____

_____

My thoughts for today:

_____

_____

_____

_____

_____

June 26th

Thought of the Day

Oftentimes when we pray for a miracle, all we really need is a renewed spirit. Once God renews your spirit, you'll be determined once again to work it out to the best of your ability or walk it out in faith until God moves on your behalf and you see success. Make your request for a renewed spirit.

My prayer for today is:

_____

_____

_____

What I will do today to go to the next level in my life:

_____

_____

_____

_____

My thoughts for today:

_____

_____

_____

_____

June 27th

Thought of the Day

Friend, you WILL BE who God says you can be. YOU WILL do every, single thing God says you can do. YOU WILL have every, single thing that God says you can have. It's up to you to walk in the will and the way of God. While doing that, push every hindrance (person or thing) out of your way. It's your season to succeed!

My prayer for today is:

_____

_____

_____

What I will do today to go to the next level in my life:

_____

_____

_____

_____

My thoughts for today:

_____

_____

_____

_____

_____

June 28th

Thought of the Day

Have you ever seen some lamenting that they can't see without their glasses and they're searching for them frantically? All the while, their glasses are on the top of their head. Once they discover that, they bring their glasses to their eyes and everything becomes clear. Similarly, in life, it's not enough to possess a gift. You have to use it to bring vision to fruition. Look at what's in front of you and go for it!

My prayer for today is:

_____

_____

_____

What I will do today to go to the next level in my life:

_____

_____

_____

_____

My thoughts for today:

_____

_____

_____

_____

_____

June 29th

Thought of the Day

There is no need to complain about a situation when it's obvious you've become content with who you are, what you're doing, how you're living, and the types of people and predicaments you always attract. All people carry the onus for themselves to initiate and sustain change. Don't like your current job? Seek the training or education needed for the opportunity you want. Don't like being out of shape? Become active. Don't like being depressed? Stop hanging out with people who depress you and find counsel in those who uplift you. Tired of being called out of your name? Don't keep answering to it.. You can't turn the page to a new day when your bookmark keeps you reading the same old passage.

My prayer for today is:

_____

_____

_____

What I will do today to go to the next level in my life:

_____

_____

_____

_____

My thoughts for today:

_____

_____

_____

_____

_____

June 30th

Thought of the Day

A relationship with God provides us with resources when we have none, rest when we feel we can't go any further, refuge when it seems we have a target on our backs, restoration when we're broken, and revival when our spirits and faith are low. Thank God that we love the Lord and that the Lord loves us. This relationship is worth more than anything imaginable. Push yourself because He is pulling for you.

My prayer for today is:

_____

_____

_____

What I will do today to go to the next level in my life:

_____

_____

_____

_____

My thoughts for today:

_____

_____

_____

_____

_____

July

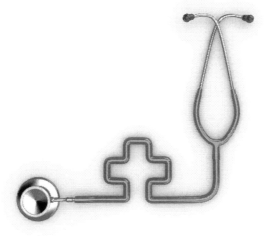

July
The Real Independence Day

Medicine

Imagine the look on my southern family's faces when I suggested that we grill vegetables for the Fourth of July! A few were okay with them as long as they sat on their plates alongside the ribs and barbequed chicken. I was good with that. At least it was a step.

We all have to make up our minds about how we eat and how active we are. Most of us can't wait until it's time for us to leave our parents' houses. Too many grown folks in one house does not work. We can't wait to be on our own. We can do what we want, including eat what we want. How many can attest that the dreaded *freshman 15* is real? It is not uncommon for many college freshmen to put on at least 15 pounds in that first year of college. While maybe all of moms' meals weren't 100% healthy, often vegetables did show up. At other times, if you didn't like what was served, your option was to just nibble on the side dishes. Talk about portion control! At those times, we secretly longed for our freedom.

Let's fast forward to when we launched out of the house. Our money was limited so dollar menus and economical pizza deals looked great. Splurging meant supersizing. The best thing was that we got exactly what we wanted every night! Who paid attention to calories? We were young. We'd work it off, right? Maybe some of us started to throw a little drinking in there. We all knew somebody in college who took up recreational activities that lead to the munchies. Sometimes we ate out of emotion. We let food become our comfort. How did we not notice that our pants were getting a little tighter? Did we miss that sweatpants were becoming our favorite attire? When you went home for a break, it was not deniable. Everybody noticed that you had put on weight. When you ate dinner, you even noticed how much you missed home cooking.

I did benefit from my father buying me a personal-size crock-pot when I was a freshman. He told me I'd better learn to throw something in that pot so it would be ready after class. Truth be told, I thought it was just a money-saving idea on his part. I think it probably was, but it was also a good health idea. I am not against the lessons that we all have to learn for ourselves. Often, we struggle to get the weight off that we happily put on until we realize the toll.

The point really is this—freedom without caution comes with a price. Life really is about balance. It's about making informed decisions. If we eat out of emotion, it may be helpful to get help for the underlying problem. If we have to have some junk food, it's best to try eating in moderation. We've got to keep our bodies active.

I have run 10 half marathons to date. One of my favorite shirts I bought at an expo says, "There will come a day when I cannot do this. Today is not that day." I love that shirt. I have to give it all I can to be the best me I can for as long as I can. Hebrews 12:1 (NIV) says, "And let us run with perseverance the race marked out for us." I believe that our physical well-being supports that. What say you, preacher?

Ministry

I've said before that our physical well-being plays a huge role in how we perform in our God-given purpose. It's really difficult at best and impossible in some cases for us to be effective and efficient in ministry when our bodies are broken down. My spiritual covering, Bishop Joseph Warren Walker III, has often quipped about how our culture feeds the preacher mac and cheese and fried chicken all the time—even late at night after a revival or convention setting. Then that preacher, without moderation and discipline, ends up huffing and puffing and feeling as if he's about to have some serious respiratory issues.

We've laughed at his presentation of these facts; but the assessment is very much valid. In my battle with weight, I can attest to the fact that the condition of our physical being has a direct correlation to how well we undertake the duties God assigns to our hands. I'm at my best in the pulpit and discharging my duties as a pastor when I'm physically active in my personal time. Conversely, the times that I haven't been very active by way of exercise and not disciplined in eating, I ended up feeling very sluggish and lethargic.

Bishop Walker spoke a truth a couple of years ago that I've never forgotten. God desires much more for us and wants to enlarge our territories to the point it blesses our lives and the lives of others immensely. However, God can't do it if we're not physically fit to handle the challenges that come with the *more* God has in store for us.

That thought has made me think, "How much of what God wants to do in my life have I missed or has been delayed because God knows physically I can't handle it right now?" That literally set me in motion. I've figured out that if I don't take care of me, then I won't be available to take care of and support others. I also might be forfeiting many blessings God has for me. Every person, even those who feel they're in great physical shape, should evaluate their physical health and seek ways to improve it. We've got a God race to run! In Hebrews 12:1-2, the race the writer refers to is centered on our faith in God and our faithfulness to God. Use your faith to believe that God can help you become a better physical, mental, emotional, and spiritual you.

July

Our prayer for this month is that you stand up for yourself. Celebrate your independence. You may sometimes feel lonely but you're never alone with God on your side. What are your goals for this month?

1.

2.

3.

July 1ˢᵗ

Thought of the Day

Aristotle said, "We are what we repeatedly do. Excellence, then, is not an act, but a habit." Have you noticed that sometimes an actor wins an Oscar for a movie that wasn't even their best movie? In those cases, the particular movie is not the only thing that is considered. It is the actor's full body of work. Don't rest after one good scene in your life. Put in the work to have a full library of excellence to your credit. Be great!

My prayer for today is:

_____

_____

_____

What I will do today to stand up for myself:

_____

_____

_____

_____

My thoughts for today:

_____

_____

_____

_____

_____

July 2nd

Thought of the Day

Chasing dreams requires one first to be a dreamer. Dreams are owned by one person at a time. Then he or she must develop a plan and determine to see the plan through. Finally, he or she must get to work without giving time or space to those who wish to simply watch, speculate, or critique. Your dreams are too important for idleness and ignorance. It's on you, through God's help, to make your dreams become reality. Now, walk it out!

My prayer for today is:

_____

_____

_____

What I will do today to stand up for myself:

_____

_____

_____

_____

My thoughts for today:

_____

_____

_____

_____

July 3rd

Thought of the Day

To increase your chances for success in living a healthy life, you have to look at the people in your circle. Different people have different levels of interest in getting and staying healthy. That's okay. I invite my friends to run with me. Some do. Even if they don't run, some will come out to walk for support. It's not one-way support either. We support each other. Even those who say I'm crazy for running still cheer me on. If there are people who hinder you or say negative things about you changing your life for the better, they are probably really not your true friends. Have you ever seen the winner of a marathon crossing the finish line? They are wearing the lightest weight clothing. They carry absolutely nothing to weigh them down. People who don't have your best interest in mind are by far the heaviest things you carry. Learn how to leave heavy things behind.

My prayer for today is:

_____

_____

_____

What I will do today to stand up for myself:

_____

_____

_____

_____

My thoughts for today:

_____

_____

_____

_____

_____

July 4th

Thought of the Day

Thomas Jefferson once said, "If you want something you've never had, you must be willing to do something you've never done." You can't want more for your life if you're not willing to put in the effort to get there. Blessings are sown into good ground. Put in the work to till the soil. You'll never know the extent of what you can do if you don't try. Today is a new day. Try a new thing.

My prayer for today is:

_____

_____

_____

What I will do today to stand up for myself:

_____

_____

_____

_____

My thoughts for today:

_____

_____

_____

_____

_____

July 5th

Thought of the Day

You don't have time to explain every thought, decision, word, move, action, and reaction to everyone around you. Friends are truly connected to you in a way that they can hear your heart without your saying a word. They don't expect you to live to please them. They are pleased to know you. You have ONE master and it's not another man or woman! Now, do YOU as God leads!

My prayer for today is:

_____

_____

_____

What I will do today to stand up for myself:

_____

_____

_____

_____

My thoughts for today:

_____

_____

_____

_____

_____

July 6th

Thought of the Day

The challenges God allows are for our development and not our destruction. Many of us are better right now because of being broken "back then." My friend, keep living and learning and the Lord will lift you at the right time, Now, make it a marvelous day!

My prayer for today is:

_____

_____

_____

What I will do today to stand up for myself:

_____

_____

_____

_____

My thoughts for today:

_____

_____

_____

_____

_____

July 7th

Thought of the Day

Life presents some days when you're down, and there is no one around to listen to you and to lift you up. That's why it's crucial that you learn how to encourage yourself in the Lord. Sometimes your own voice is the only one needed. You know how we don't like to hear our own voices on recordings? We're focused on what it sounds like but do we listen to what we're saying. Strong words of positivity can smooth out the tone. Lift your own voice and encourage yourself to be blessed!

My prayer for today is:

_____

_____

_____

What I will do today to stand up for myself:

_____

_____

_____

_____

My thoughts for today:

_____

_____

_____

_____

_____

July 8th

Thought of the Day

To be a true difference-maker, one's approach and attitude, tone and tenor, as well as perspective, patience, and processes often differ greatly from others. Be okay with that! At the end of the day, it's all about producing meaningful results and great successes with dignity, character, integrity, humility, and respect still being your hallmarks.

My prayer for today is:

_____

_____

_____

What I will do today to stand up for myself:

_____

_____

_____

My thoughts for today:

_____

_____

_____

_____

July 9th

Thought of the Day

I am a firm believer that God, at times, meticulously places some of life's mountains in front of us not to conquer us but to teach us to develop the mentality to challenge our challenges. Have a mind to be a mountain climber! Better yet, use your faith and become a mountain mover!

My prayer for today is:

_____

_____

_____

What I will do today to stand up for myself:

_____

_____

_____

_____

My thoughts for today:

_____

_____

_____

_____

July 10th

Thought of the Day

The Little Engine That Could kept encouraging himself as he climbed a mighty steep hill. We should try to do the same by adopting his words no matter what we face. Look at the problem, issue, situation, or difficult task and with a heart of faith say, "I think I can! I think I can!" Then remember God's on your side. Believe in yourself even more! That'll lead you to change the wording a bit to "I KNOW I can!"

My prayer for today is:

_____

_____

_____

What I will do today to stand up for myself:

_____

_____

_____

_____

My thoughts for today:

_____

_____

_____

_____

July 11th

Thought of the Day

Some people will become adversarial when you won't feed their attention-getting and apathy about making their own situations better! Be cool with it and keep moving. People who want to get better may ask to lean on you for support, but they won't ask you to carry them.

My prayer for today is:

_____

_____

_____

What I will do today to stand up for myself:

_____

_____

_____

_____

My thoughts for today:

_____

_____

_____

_____

_____

July 12th

Thoughts of the Day

Doing the right thing and standing for what is right may cost us some "friends" and popularity. However, I'll take that as opposed to losing my joy, peace of mind, character, integrity, and close connection to God. Don't compromise your standards just to stand with those who aren't standing for anything positive.

My prayer for today is:

_____

_____

_____

What I will do today to stand up for myself:

_____

_____

_____

My thoughts for today:

_____

_____

_____

_____

_____

July 13th

Thought of the Day

We must understand that there will be those who will never understand our faith walk. However, never stop walking just to appease those content to stand still. It's your journey that will lead to your joy. Therefore, keeping following Jesus even if means others will keep asking why, when, where, and how. Keep the faith!

My prayer for today is:

_____

_____

_____

What I will do today to stand up for myself:

_____

_____

_____

_____

My thoughts for today:

_____

_____

_____

_____

_____

July 14th

Thought of the Day

Keep in mind that no one can pray you through something that you're comfortable and complacent being in. Before asking others to stand in agreement with you that "God will move," be sure you're ready to move and do everything necessary to precipitate progress! God steps in for those ready to step forward. Put on your stepping shoes today!

My prayer for today is:

_____

_____

_____

What I will do today to stand up for myself:

_____

_____

_____

_____

My thoughts for today:

_____

_____

_____

_____

_____

July 15th

Thought of the Day

Social media was used to influence a presidential election. Seeds of deception were planted that sprouted everywhere. The CEOs of the social media companies were called before Congress to testify and asked how they allowed it to happen. They had some responsibility for the rules of their platform that may not have been secure enough. We have the ultimate responsibility to practice discernment. We can't fall for anything. Turn to facts to stamp out fiction. Turn to faith when the facts look discouraging. Don't be influenced. Be informed.

My prayer for today is:

_____

_____

_____

What I will do today to stand up for myself:

_____

_____

_____

_____

My thoughts for today:

_____

_____

_____

_____

_____

July 16th

Thought of the Day

You must remember that if excellence is what you demand of yourself, demand it also of those in your circle. Demand it of anything you're connected to. Oftentimes you'll receive more criticism than compliments. Be okay with that. Don't lessen yourself to average just to be accepted. Eagles soar high but they soar alone. Fly high even if you have to soar alone.

My prayer for today is:

_____

_____

_____

What I will do today to stand up for myself:

_____

_____

_____

My thoughts for today:

_____

_____

_____

_____

July 17th

Thought of the Day

Nike has trademarked the phrase "just do it." I think the reason it resonates with so many of us is that it resonates with faith. With faith, you can visualize yourself past your current situation, eventually enjoying victory over the situation. You can push yourself further. You can't conquer that wellness journey, that exercise journey, or any of life's journeys if you refuse to try. You have to speak to yourself to take the leap. Just do it!

My prayer for today is:

_____

_____

_____

What I will do today to stand up for myself:

_____

_____

_____

_____

My thoughts for today:

_____

_____

_____

_____

_____

July 18th

Thought of the Day

Never apologize for the success, blessings, prosperity, or productivity that the Lord has allowed you to enjoy. After all, very few people know the processes, pain, and pressure you endured to be where you are now. If you gave up your blessings, they would be glad to take them! God doesn't have a limit on blessings. Instead of letting anyone bring you down, encourage them to come up. If they don't want to make the trip, wish them well.

My prayer for today is:

_____

_____

_____

What I will do today to stand up for myself:

_____

_____

_____

My thoughts for today:

_____

_____

_____

_____

July 19th

Thought of the Day

Something being easy doesn't always equate to it being right. Likewise, something being difficult doesn't always equate to it being wrong. God often uses difficulties as developmental tools to produce the character and commitment necessary to make your dreams become reality. So it's best you learn to press your way through tough times.

My prayer for today is:

_____

_____

_____

What I will do today to stand up for myself:

_____

_____

_____

_____

My thoughts for today:

_____

_____

_____

_____

_____

July 20th

Thought of the Day

Come to grips with the fact that there are some people who will never mature to the point of being focused and productive. Be okay with proceeding, progressing, and producing in your life while they continue to specialize in trivial pettiness in their lives. Don't be tied or turned by those whose heads and hearts are twisted. Go forward on this favored day!

My prayer for today is:

_____

_____

_____

What I will do today to stand up for myself:

_____

_____

_____

_____

My thoughts for today:

_____

_____

_____

_____

_____

July 21st

Thought of the Day

Failures and disappointments will either teach us and lead us into our future or tie us and lock us into our past. We must make the conscious decision if we're going to stay or go. Let's go!

My prayer for today is:

_____

_____

_____

What I will do today to stand up for myself:

_____

_____

_____

_____

My thoughts for today:

_____

_____

_____

_____

_____

July 22nd

Thought of the Day

One bad spark plug can kill your entire engine. In that case, you remove the plug, replace the plug, restart the car, and keep it moving. Likewise, one person with a bad attitude and negative perspective can kill your focus, your dreams, your joy, your excitement, and your motivation. Treat them like a spark plug. Remove them from your company, replace them with someone who believes in you and sees the best, restart your life, and keep it moving.

My prayer for today is:

_____

_____

_____

What I will do today to stand up for myself:

_____

_____

_____

My thoughts for today:

_____

_____

_____

_____

July 23rd

Thought of the Day

If you follow football, you may have heard that Andrew Luck, the quarterback of the Indianapolis Colts, stunned fans everywhere by suddenly retiring seemingly out of the blue at the age of 29. He chose to walk away from hundreds of millions of dollars. The constant injuries had dulled his love of the game. He decided his health and his family were more important. It just goes to show that some things that look like they are good TO you may not be good FOR you. Deep down, we know this. It's about having the strength to walk away. Sometimes we have to be sick and tired of being sick and tired before we can leave a situation. Choose to leave before the situation takes too much of your energy—energy you could be applying toward a greater cause.

My prayer for today is:

_____

_____

_____

What I will do today to stand up for myself:

_____

_____

_____

_____

My thoughts for today:

_____

_____

_____

_____

_____

July 24th

Thought of the Day

When you are comfortable being yourself, it doesn't make you uncomfortable when other people don't understand you or don't want to understand you. Be cool with having a small circle. After all, the winner's circle rarely has multiple pedestals. Thank God that you are you.

My prayer for today is:

_____

_____

_____

What I will do today to stand up for myself:

_____

_____

_____

_____

My thoughts for today:

_____

_____

_____

_____

_____

July 25th

Thought of the Day

At some point you have to move on. When you've truly done that, you don't spend time, money, effort, texts, calls, emails, Facebook posts, etc., justifying, validating, spotlighting, and defending. When you've truly moved on, your mind and your mouth reset and refocus. Your spirit is renewed. Then you can worship, work, and watch God work on your behalf. Insecurity yields to inspiration and anxiety yields to anticipation of what will BE rather than what WAS. Let it go. Let it be. Then look forward and not behind.

My prayer for today is:

_____

_____

_____

What I will do today to stand up for myself:

_____

_____

_____

_____

My thoughts for today:

_____

_____

_____

_____

July 26th

Thought of the Day

Our dad has the ultimate gift of willpower. After he had been a long-time smoker, he decided one day the habit was too costly. He quit cold turkey. He examined the facts and made a change. We know faith trumps facts, but I believe facts can show you where to focus your faith. Be intentional on your faith walk today!

My prayer for today is:

_____

_____

_____

What I will do today to stand up for myself:

_____

_____

_____

_____

My thoughts for today:

_____

_____

_____

_____

July 27th

Thought of the Day

Remember, God doesn't always just do things for us and give things to us. Sometimes He puts the blessing in front of us and gives us the responsibility to press and produce in order to get the blessings. Exercising your faith and exhausting your efforts are key principles in being who God would have you to be, doing what God would have you to do, and having what God would have you to have. Focus forward on this favored day.

My prayer for today is:

_____

_____

_____

What I will do today to stand up for myself:

_____

_____

_____

My thoughts for today:

_____

_____

_____

_____

July 28th

Thought of the Day

Sometimes God will allow you to get to the end of your rope so you'll finally let go of the rope and grab His hand. God wants to keep and cover you. First, you must be and stay connected to Him. He can and will help you get to the top of your mountain.

My prayer for today is:

_____

_____

_____

What I will do today to stand up for myself:

_____

_____

_____

_____

My thoughts for today:

_____

_____

_____

_____

_____

July 29th

Thought of the Day

You will never set secure boundaries in your life if first you're not honest about your insecurities and vulnerabilities. Sometimes being strong means not putting yourself in situations that make you tempted to do something you shouldn't. It's about not being around people who influence you to do things the old you used to do. Sometimes, it's avoiding situations that are unhealthy. Know what you need to stay away from to keep on the right track!

My prayer for today is:

_____

_____

_____

What I will do today to stand up for myself:

_____

_____

_____

My thoughts for today:

_____

_____

_____

_____

July 30th

Thought of the Day

Sometimes prayer and faith are all you have. Don't fret! This spiritual dynamic duo is most often all you need. Prayer and faith touch the heart of God and ultimately move the hand of God. So, friend, pray in faith and watch God move!

My prayer for today is:

_____

_____

_____

What I will do today to stand up for myself:

_____

_____

_____

_____

My thoughts for today:

_____

_____

_____

_____

_____

July 31st

Thought of the Day

I always tell my son when he is driving somewhere or traveling to let me know when he gets there. He thinks he's too grown and that I'm being overprotective. I explain to him that I know he's capable of getting to his destination by himself. However, if something unusual happens and he is unable to call or text me, he should be comforted in knowing that his Mama will do everything in her power to find him and get him to safety. That only works if our communication is consistent even in those times where there is no trouble. God made you to stand on your own but you need to stay connected to Him even when times are good. And when the bad days roll around, you'll be comforted in knowing your help is on the way.

My prayer for today is:

_____

_____

_____

What I will do today to stand up for myself:

_____

_____

_____

_____

My thoughts for today:

_____

_____

_____

_____

_____

August

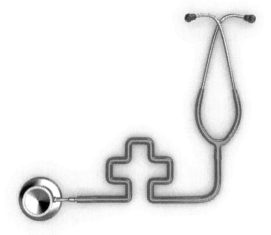

August
Summertime – And Sometimes the Living Ain't Easy

Medicine

I try to stay fit. As I mentioned, I have run half marathons. I have worked with a personal trainer for 7 years now (shout-out to Gerell Webb). Before some of you roll your eyes and say that I have it easy because I have a personal trainer, I have to ask, "Have you met a personal trainer?" My favorite saying during workouts is, "Help me, Father." I mean it! There is nothing easy about that uphill running my trainer has me do. There is nothing easy when I forget to breathe during those evil push-ups that cause sweat to pool on the floor from my forehead. I assure you. If you saw me struggling to do pull-ups, you would wonder if a blood vessel was going to burst in my head. And burpees! I think there is an illustration of a burpee next to *torture* in the dictionary. A trainer's job is to design a plan; but it's my job to execute it.

My trainer likes to tell the story of when we first started training. The first time we trained, he was nice and eased me into things. I even had on a little face powder and lip-gloss and thought I still looked cute at the end of the workout. The second time we trained, it was at my house. He taught me how to use things in my house for exercise purposes versus my feeling the need to join a gym. By the time he left, my little face power was all over my shirt from the sweat. I locked the door behind him and collapsed on the floor. I couldn't move. A wave of nausea finally forced me to jump up and run to the bathroom. I seriously contemplated quitting. I said bad things about my trainer. I thought God would even understand why.

However, with strokes running in my family, I was determined to have that generational curse end with me. That's why I connected with a trainer. I wanted that motivation and accountability to make sure that trend didn't continue with me. I started praying earnestly over the situation. I prayed to God that I wouldn't die during the training and that I wouldn't kill my trainer during the sessions.

The next time I saw my trainer, even though I had prayed for 30 full minutes before seeing him, he looked at me and asked, "Are you okay?" I told him with a pretty intense face that every time I even thought of him, I wanted to throw up. That was the truth. Seven years later, I'm still with him. I never wear face powder now because I am no longer trying to be cute. I come to fight. Every time I think I've mastered something, he ups the stakes and makes the workout harder so I always have to dig deep. Why do I stay with him? It's like someone said, "If you stay ready, you don't have to get ready."

I also truly liken working out to the Christian journey. First of all, I take it one day at a time. It's not easy, but it doesn't mean it's not worth it. I am hungry for positive change. If I can do it, others in my family can too. My trainer never tells me I can't eat what I want but he does remind me that when I eat junk, I will pay for it. In other words, there are consequences to our actions.

You don't have to have a trainer, but I urge you to have an accountability partner. Even if you are a loner, this is one place where you might benefit from trying something new. Not only can you be motivated by someone else but perhaps you can be the motivation he or she needs. Jesus often sent the disciples out in two's, didn't he, preacher?

Ministry

He did. Among other things, in numerology the number two signifies "an adequate witness" and "needed support." One of the greatest misnomers ever perpetuated is that we don't need anyone else. It's not true. I believe that God often anoints people to be exactly what other people need in certain seasons of their lives. Consider 2 Kings 5 when Naaman wanted to be healed of leprosy. That brother got really upset when he made it to Elisha's house, and the prophet sent a servant outside to tell him to go dip in the Jordan River seven times. Naaman thought the least Elisha could do is come outside, wave his hand over him, and say a prayer. Naaman was in a bad mental space. His attitude was horrible. However, he was surrounded by some people who told him the truth. They basically said, "Best you worry about compliance rather than ceremony. You want to be healed. So go on and dip yourself in Jordan." Naaman gathered his senses, dipped seven times, and ended up healed. Thank God, he had some folks hold him accountable.

That's exactly what we need for every facet of our lives. We should embrace godly connections with people who will hold us accountable. Whether it's spiritually, physically, emotionally, financially, professionally, or otherwise, accountability partners—people who God sends—will help keep us focused in our present while embracing our future goals.

Accountability partners are often true friends. However, they're not to always agree with us. They're not to pacify us. They're not to lie to us. They're not to enable us. In fact, there are times that those in our circles should love us enough to put our egos in check. They should love us enough to snatch us out of our pity parties. They should love us enough to possibly even hurt our feelings now so we'll be better off later. At day's end, those God sends to connect to us will always add to our lives and not take away. They'll be builders. They'll be, as Dr. Sam Chand says, "ladder holders" who will steady life's ladders for us so we can climb higher.

Ask God for true friends. Ask God for true accountability partners. Then ask Him for the heart, mind, and emotional balance to receive how He wants to impact and influence your life through them.

August

Our hope for you this month is that when times get hard, your determination to overcome strengthens. What are your goals for this month?

1.

2.

3.

August 1st

Thought of the Day

I can't tell you how many remixes I've done of *One Day at a Time*. I might throw in some specific references to what I'm going through at the time but the chorus remains the same. "One day at a time, sweet Jesus. That's all I'm asking from you. Give me the strength to do every day what I have to do. Yesterday's gone, sweet Jesus, and tomorrow may never be mine. So for my sake, teach me to take one day at a time." All I can say after that is, Amen!

My prayer for today is:

_____

_____

_____

What I will do today to strengthen myself:

_____

_____

_____

My thoughts for today:

_____

_____

_____

_____

_____

August 2nd

Thought of the Day

When I run, I know that miles 1 and 2 are extremely challenging for me. Even after I get in a rhythm of training and my endurance has improved, the first couple of miles are still hard for me. Usually at miles 3 and 4, I start to feel good. In the beginning, I always wanted to give up as early as the first mile. Over time, I learned to tell myself, "Know what you know." I know it starts off hard and then it gets better. Much of running is mental. The reason I can push through the initial challenge now is that I know for sure that it will get better. Even if you're going through a difficult situation; call on what you know. "Weeping endures for a night, but joy comes in the morning" (Psalm 30:5).

My prayer for today is:

_____

_____

_____

What I will do today to strengthen myself:

_____

_____

_____

_____

My thoughts for today:

_____

_____

_____

_____

August 3rd

Thought of the Day

"Why me?" That's what we often wonder when bad things happen. That's a question we ask in our flesh. Let's answer it with our faith by remembering that the rain falls on the just and the unjust. God allowed Job to be challenged and he gave him a double reward for his trouble. Has God allowed this because He knows you can weather the storm and others will bear witness to it? This too will pass. You'll be stronger on the other side. God allows nothing to happen that you and He together cannot handle.

My prayer for today is:

_____

_____

_____

What I will do today to strengthen myself:

_____

_____

_____

My thoughts for today:

_____

_____

_____

_____

August 4th

Thought of the Day

I am paraphrasing Bishop Joseph Warren Walker, III who said, "Peace is not the absence of storms, but it is learning how to react in the midst of the storms." Peace doesn't just come to you. It takes active steps to achieve it. Have you ever gone to the grocery store in the south when there is a weather forecast of snow? The bread and milk shelves are always empty! I'll be honest, I'm not sure why bread and milk are the staples of choice. The point is to have things you can consume if you can't get out and you lose electrical power. It takes being hungry and cold once to make you be prepared for it the next time. Learn from your storm and be ready to withstand it the next time.

My prayer for today is:

_____

_____

_____

What I will do today to strengthen myself:

_____

_____

_____

_____

My thoughts for today:

_____

_____

_____

_____

August 5th

Thought of the Day

If you are serious about making a change, let people you trust know. It adds accountability. You can share your walks or runs, as well as what you eat, through apps. Word of mouth works also. My dad is notorious for asking me when I'm about to do a race and if I plan to do better. As much as he's asking me, he's also telling me I should strive to keep improving. I have some great race days! Sometimes I'm just glad I finished. Either way, I hear Dad's voice asking me if I'm pushing to do better. That gives me an extra boost. At the end of the race, I want to be able to tell him that I absolutely did my best. Will you be able to tell your Father you did your best?

My prayer for today is:

_____

_____

_____

What I will do today to strengthen myself:

_____

_____

_____

_____

My thoughts for today:

_____

_____

_____

_____

August 6th

Thought of the Day

Most of us are afraid of pain. Take childbirth as an example. Some women say they forget the pain when they see their beautiful babies. I can tell you I definitely did not forget the pain from childbirth, but my son constantly reminds me it was worth the pain. No life is free from pain. We can't forget that good can come on the other side of pain. Don't expend your energy running from the pain. Instead, use that energy to run through it to the other side.

My prayer for today is:

_____

_____

_____

What I will do today to strengthen myself:

_____

_____

_____

My thoughts for today:

_____

_____

_____

_____

August 7th

Thought of the Day

Why do we wait to get ready when trouble is already upon us? Why do we wait to exercise after we've already gained weight? Why do we wait to get mental health help when our depression has gotten so bad that we can't get out of bed? Being proactive is practicing wisdom. John F. Kennedy once said, "The time to repair the roof is when the sun is shining." As the saying goes, "You don't have to get ready if you stay ready."

My prayer for today is:

_____

_____

_____

What I will do today to strengthen myself:

_____

_____

_____

_____

My thoughts for today:

_____

_____

_____

_____

August 8th

Thought of the Day

Refuse to be reluctant to tell and show others how God has blessed you. Your humble witness of His goodness to you and how you give God glory may be the encouragement someone needs to persevere until God works on their behalf. They need to know the One who blessed you desires to bless them as well. Be the best advertisement of God's blessings today!

My prayer for today is:

_____

_____

_____

What I will do today to strengthen myself:

_____

_____

_____

_____

My thoughts for today:

_____

_____

_____

_____

_____

August 9th

Thought of the Day

Deliverance from something or someone most often IS NOT sudden. Instead, it's a gradual process. It often takes baby steps for an individual to be healed, be made whole, get past something traumatic, and see the changes he or she desperately wants and needs. So don't be discouraged if things don't change or get better in an instant. Instead, concentrate on getting and being just a little bit better today than yesterday. Learn to celebrate small steps of success.

My prayer for today is:

_____

_____

_____

What I will do today to strengthen myself:

_____

_____

_____

_____

My thoughts for today:

_____

_____

_____

_____

_____

August 10th

Thought of the Day

Sometimes God won't allow your struggles and pain to remain private no matter how hard you try. That's so when He blesses you, changes your situation, defends you, heals you, and open doors for you, the public will have to testify of His ability, grace, love, and power. You're a walking, talking billboard for how the Lord blesses those who trust Him.

My prayer for today is:

_____

_____

_____

What I will do today to strengthen myself:

_____

_____

_____

_____

My thoughts for today:

_____

_____

_____

_____

_____

August 11th

Thought of the Day

The way to make it through today is to remember the One who has kept you, protected you, provided for you, sustained you, and been there for you all of the other days of your life. Different day. Same God.

My prayer for today is:

_____

_____

_____

What I will do today to strengthen myself:

_____

_____

_____

_____

My thoughts for today:

_____

_____

_____

_____

_____

August 12ᵗʰ

Thought of the Day

Being focused for the day begins with first telling God "THANK YOU" for allowing you to see a new day. Because we all are flawed and undeserving of God's goodness, we should be grateful that grace and mercy made the difference on our behalf. Make it a marvelous day!

My prayer for today is:

_____

_____

_____

What I will do today to strengthen myself:

_____

_____

_____

My thoughts for today:

_____

_____

_____

_____

_____

August 13th

Thought of the Day

Seven words to lift your spirits and hopes by faith GOD IS WORKING IT OUT RIGHT NOW! So give God praise now for what He's in the process of doing. Thank Him while He's turning circumstances around for you!

My prayer for today is:

_____

_____

_____

What I will do today to strengthen myself:

_____

_____

_____

_____

My thoughts for today:

_____

_____

_____

_____

_____

August 14th

Thought of the Day

In life you're going to win some and you're going to lose some. In all of them, make sure you're prepared, positive, confident, and courageous. If not, you've lost before you even begin.

My prayer for today is:

_____

_____

_____

What I will do today to strengthen myself:

_____

_____

_____

My thoughts for today:

_____

_____

_____

_____

August 15th

Thought of the Day

There are no limits when it comes to what God can do. Therefore, don't limit your hopes and dreams. Put in the work and watch God work. As the song *He's Able* says, "Don't give up on God because He won't give up on you."

My prayer for today is:

_____

_____

_____

What I will do today to strengthen myself:

_____

_____

_____

My thoughts for today:

_____

_____

_____

_____

August 16th

Thought of the Day

Keep holding on to God's powerful hand. His hand is big enough to support you no matter the challenge, strong and mighty enough to fight for you no matter the giants you face, and gentle enough to love, comfort, and keep you no matter the test and trial.

My prayer for today is:

_____

_____

_____

What I will do today to strengthen myself:

_____

_____

_____

My thoughts for today:

_____

_____

_____

_____

August 17th

Thought of the Day

Sometimes we all just need to press pause on our hectic lives. I think one of the reasons Psalm 23 is one of the most familiar passages in the Bible is because reading it immediately summons peaceful imagery in the mind's eye and brings comfort to the soul. Find time to take rest in knowing that the Lord is your shepherd.

My prayer for today is:

_____

_____

_____

What I will do today to strengthen myself:

_____

_____

_____

_____

My thoughts for today:

_____

_____

_____

_____

_____

August 18th

Thought of the Day

Prayer only works when your prayers are born out of the belief that God will hear your plea, heal your pain, and help in your predicament. In other words, if you're going to call God, then be confident God will come when, where, and how you need Him most. Ask, knowing you will receive.

My prayer for today is:

_____

_____

_____

What I will do today to strengthen myself:

_____

_____

_____

_____

My thoughts for today:

_____

_____

_____

_____

August 19th

Thought of the Day

James Baldwin said, "Not everything that is faced can be changed, but nothing can be changed until it is faced." Sometimes we avoid challenges because they seem insurmountable. We even think we might be doing a good job in denying the existence of our problems until we realize they are keeping us from sleeping at night. An unfaced problem seems even bigger than it is because our anxiety mounts up on top of it. Pray for strength to face the challenge that stands in your way. You owe it to yourself to find out if your path is over the mountain or around it.

My prayer for today is:

_____

_____

_____

What I will do today to strengthen myself:

_____

_____

_____

_____

My thoughts for today:

_____

_____

_____

_____

_____

August 20th

Thought of the Day

Atlanta Braves lead-off hitter Ronald Acuna, Jr. was intentionally hit by the Florida Marlins pitcher on his first pitch of a game in 2018. Acuna was hit so hard and appeared so badly hurt that he immediately left the game. He also left many to wonder if he'd return to the line-up in weeks. Well, one day after being drilled by the enemy, Acuna was back in the batter's box, still hurting, but refusing to be defeated. Friend, the enemy hit you pretty hard, huh? People doubt your return, huh? Although you're still hurting, keep fighting. Get back in the batter's box and get back to winning.

My prayer for today is:

_____

_____

_____

What I will do today to strengthen myself:

_____

_____

_____

My thoughts for today:

_____

_____

_____

_____

August 21ˢᵗ

Thought of the Day

God never promised us that every day and everything would be easy. Let's have heart. Let's hold our heads up. And let's meet our challenges head-on. Sometimes the greatest blessings are just on the other side of what you thought was your breaking point.

My prayer for today is:

_____

_____

_____

What I will do today to strengthen myself:

_____

_____

_____

My thoughts for today:

_____

_____

_____

_____

August 22nd

Thought of the Day

Many of us need to stop pretending like we never make mistakes. There are times we need to be transparent about our trials and how God moved to turn our lives around. In this season, "religion" will not win people to Christ. However, our transparency in sharing the reality that we've had some major mess-ups that God covered with grace and mercy may be the very thing that brings others hope and closer to Christ. Tell it like it is!

My prayer for today is:

_____

_____

_____

What I will do today to strengthen myself:

_____

_____

_____

My thoughts for today:

_____

_____

_____

_____

_____

August 23rd

Thought of the Day

You'll never recover from the hurt and pain if you choose to reside in that spiritual, mental, and emotional low place. Recovery and restoration begin the moment you refuse to worry, wallow, and whine. Our mother has had knee replacement surgery. She can tell you that it's not long after the surgery that the surgeon wants you up and walking, even if you have some pain. The pain will subside quicker if you work through it. The joint will heal better if you put it through it's normal range of motion as soon as possible. You don't want it to get stiff and stuck in place. Healing doesn't just happen. It requires your participation. Get up! Get going!

My prayer for today is:

_____

_____

_____

What I will do today to strengthen myself:

_____

_____

_____

_____

My thoughts for today:

_____

_____

_____

_____

_____

August 24th

Thought of the Day

Many people lose long before a contest or event is over or before a situation is resolved. If your mind can't conceive "good success" and your heart doesn't believe you'll win or overcome, you lost the moment you created and fed doubts. Believe and achieve on this BLESSED day.

My prayer for today is:

_____

_____

_____

What I will do today to strengthen myself:

_____

_____

_____

_____

My thoughts for today:

_____

_____

_____

_____

_____

August 25th

Thought of the Day

Often, too much emphasis is put on finishing first and finishing with all the accolades. However, the most important thing for some people is just FINISHING. Sometimes one can endure so much along life's journey that just finishing is a major victory. Friend, no matter what life throws your way, set your mind and heart to finish strong and well in everything you endeavor!

My prayer for today is:

_____

_____

_____

What I will do today to strengthen myself:

_____

_____

_____

_____

My thoughts for today:

_____

_____

_____

_____

_____

August 26th

Thought of the Day

I'm reminded of something my friend Pastor Chris Wimberly said during our revival meetings. He had a word of encouragement for everyone who felt beaten and broken by life and by people. He said, "You've got to keep living. You've got to keep doing your best. You can't give up. You can't call it quits. Just remember that broken crayons still color." That's your word, my friend. There is still promise and potential for your life despite the pain and pressure coming your way. No matter the circumstance, "keep coloring."

My prayer for today is:

_____

_____

_____

What I will do today to strengthen myself:

_____

_____

_____

_____

My thoughts for today:

_____

_____

_____

_____

August 27th

Thought of the Day

Today, many people will have their eyes to the sky whether looking for storms, peaks of sunshine,, or even signs of help from Heaven. The good news is that EVERY DAY the One who reigns over the earth and skies has His eyes on you! We serve a BIG God who is still so intimate and close to us that He cares for us, covers us, and keeps us when meteorological storms AND life's storms rage. He sees you!

My prayer for today is:

_____

_____

_____

What I will do today to strengthen myself:

_____

_____

_____

_____

My thoughts for today:

_____

_____

_____

_____

_____

August 28th

Thought of the Day

Always remember that the times we deem as "bad" often serve as the perfect backdrop for our mighty good and powerful God to assess our situations, assist us, and see us through. You may "go through" it, but God will get you through it, so He can receive the glory. That said, thank Him now for what He's about to do. Make it a great day, my friend!

My prayer for today is:

_____

_____

_____

What I will do today to strengthen myself:

_____

_____

_____

My thoughts for today:

_____

_____

_____

_____

August 29th

Thought of the Day

Too often we focus on "what could go wrong" rather than on the One "who makes things right." The Bible says, "Therefore, do not worry about tomorrow, for tomorrow will worry about itself" (Matthew 6:34, NIV). Each day has enough trouble of its own. God will never call you to it and not see you through it!

My prayer for today is:

_____

_____

_____

What I will do today to strengthen myself:

_____

_____

_____

My thoughts for today:

_____

_____

_____

_____

August 30th

Thought of the Day

Never give people total access to your life when it is apparent they lack discipline, maturity, order, spiritual growth, and focus to their lives. It is okay to have a close, closed circle of friends. Be intimate only with those who are truly into God and into you. True friends share joys and tears. They have many things in common but celebrate each other's differences. They push each other to accomplish their goals. To have good friends, you have to be a good friend. I firmly believe good friends are good for your mental health.

My prayer for today is:

_____

_____

_____

What I will do today to strengthen myself:

_____

_____

_____

My thoughts for today:

_____

_____

_____

_____

August 31st

Thought of the Day

There is one blessing from God that we rarely talk about but looms so important: the blessing of non-exposure. Aren't you glad that our Father loves us so much that He hasn't made public every mistake and misdeed done in private? This is the essence of His grace and mercy. #nohashtag #thismistakewillnotbepublic

My prayer for today is:

_____

_____

_____

What I will do today to strengthen myself:

_____

_____

_____

_____

My thoughts for today:

_____

_____

_____

_____

_____

September

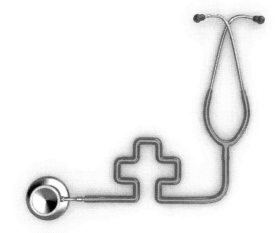

September
Fall Transitions

Medicine

Fall is my favorite season. Trees begin to let go of their green leaves in exchange for the warm orange, red, and yellow leaves of autumn. We start to pull out our sweaters and boots. Sometimes, it feels like summer struggles to give up its hold by interrupting the coolness with a few more hot days. In other words, transitions take time. That applies to transitions within our lives as well. We sometimes face struggles as we move into a new season. Metaphorically speaking, fall issues us into a more mature time in our lives. We can embrace that or we can become fearful of the winter that we know is coming next. If fear grips us, it can impact other decisions in our lives.

For example, do we commit to a healthy lifestyle when we know changes can happen to our bodies with age? I believe that we cannot be resigned to thinking that we can't positively influence how we age. I've heard people say eating healthy may make them live longer, but the food is boring and bland. On the other hand, they know unhealthy food is not good for them, but maybe it's better to be overweight and happy. The question really becomes, are they happy in the moment when they're eating and unhappy the rest of the time because of the consequences of that eating? That leads to another question. Does food fill a void? If so, what is it? Should you get help for what may be affecting you emotionally, or do you continue to try to self-medicate with food?

Other times, it may feel like we are thrust into transitions. It could be that we are facing a new life situation. Sometimes situations occur where we are suddenly hit with grief or maybe we're facing discontent with our current jobs. We know seasons change but we don't expect them overnight. We can't become dormant like the plants that wait to bloom again in the spring. Fall should be a beautiful time, and we have to keep growing through it. If you have to ask yourself the question over and over, if you need help to cope or to help guide you through the transition, I believe you already know the answer. We love to say, "The struggle is real." That preaches right there! When you know the struggle is real, get real about addressing the struggle. Paul wrote that he learned to be content. He didn't mean to give up in your situation, did he, preacher?

Ministry

No, not at all. When Paul wrote about his contentment in Philippians 4:10-12, he rejoiced in the fact that people at Philippi had begun caring for him again. In this text, Paul relayed his plight of

293

knowing the reality of having a lot materially and the reality of having little materially. He knew how to be on top of the world. He also knew the feeling of the world seemingly being on top of him. He stated in verse 11: "For I have learned in whatsoever state I am, therewith to be content." Paul's declaration of contentment wasn't indicative of him pressing pause on his ministry. All Paul was really saying was, in essence, "No matter what state I find myself in, I've learned to have a settled mind and a settled spirit."

You may wonder how Paul could be so calm and confident. Well, Philippians 4:13 says it all: "I can do all things through Christ which strengtheneth me." Paul testified that with God there are no limits. Yes, things can go wrong. Yes, things can go sideways. However, it's not over as long as God is still on the throne. I love to say, "It is what it is. But it's not what it's going to be." We must look at life and all life presents through the prism of faith that allows us to see better days even while experiencing what feels like our worst days.

That principle applies to every facet of our lives as well. In health, the facts may be that you are obese. The facts may be that you have some respiratory concerns. The facts may be that your senses are diminishing. The facts may be that there are a myriad of things wrong in your body. However, you can't just sit and say, "Oh well. That's just how life goes." No, in many instances, you have the ability to improve your situation through some lifestyle changes, some hard decisions, and some hard work. Whether it's a physical ailment or mental concern, there is help available.

First, resolve that the current plight is not the end of your story. Secondly, you must seek God and also seek wisdom from trusted people on how you should address, confront, and, in many cases, ultimately conquer what concerns you. However, rest assured of one thing: resting in current miseries will never bring needed and wanted change.

September

Our prayer for you this month is that you embrace the transitions in your life and make them beautiful new seasons. What are your goals for this month?

1.

2.

3.

September 1st

Thought of the Day

Do you ever watch football? Sometimes, your team will try a play that didn't work and then they line up to try the very same play the next time. If you're like me, you might be thinking, why in the world would they do that? To your surprise, the next time, the play works! What was the difference? It may have been that the play wasn't the problem. It may have been that the execution wasn't exactly what it should have been. As in life, don't give up on doing the right thing even when the path to the right thing may have once gone wrong.

My prayer for today is:

_____

_____

_____

What I will do today to embrace this season in my life:

_____

_____

_____

_____

My thoughts for today:

_____

_____

_____

_____

September 2nd

Thought of the Day

Too often we anticipate the next blessing and get frustrated when it doesn't come as soon as we'd like. All the while we've yet to stop and truly thank God for what He's already done and for what He's doing currently.

My prayer for today is:

_____

_____

_____

What I will do today to embrace this season in my life:

_____

_____

_____

_____

My thoughts for today:

_____

_____

_____

_____

_____

September 3rd

Thought of the Day

When life is like a roller coaster, do what you'd do on a real roller coaster. Hang on, hold on, handle the highs and lows, keep it together in the winding curves, and even holler and scream! All the while, remember that God is ultimately in control. Before the wild ride began, He made sure that you were safe and secure in Him. That means sooner or later He'll straighten your path and bring you to a peaceful rest. Make it a MARVELOUS day, my friend!

My prayer for today is:

_____

_____

_____

What I will do today to embrace this season in my life:

_____

_____

_____

_____

My thoughts for today:

_____

_____

_____

_____

_____

September 4th

Thought of the Day

Faith allows one to see oneself in the next season of life while striving, sometimes struggling, and taking careful, calculated steps in the current season of life. It's simple. Right now, you are where you are in your life. But it's not where you're going to be!

My prayer for today is:

_____

_____

_____

What I will do today to embrace this season in my life:

_____

_____

_____

_____

My thoughts for today:

_____

_____

_____

_____

_____

September 5th

Thought of the Day

Never let frustration be the fuel that shapes your actions, ambitions, emotions, or thinking. It will almost always lead you to a place where there is no peace or positive productivity. Sometimes prayer, a deep breath, and doing nothing for a moment is the antidote for frustration that will get you back on the right track.

My prayer for today is:

_____

_____

_____

What I will do today to embrace this season in my life:

_____

_____

_____

_____

My thoughts for today:

_____

_____

_____

_____

_____

September 6th

Thought of the Day

This may come as a complete surprise to you, but today I want to encourage you to QUIT! You read it right. I want you to QUIT! Resolve today to QUIT agonizing over what's not important. QUIT beating yourself up over what God has forgiven. QUIT continuing to allow people to dictate your dreams. QUIT complaining as if God hasn't been good to you. QUIT draining yourself trying to help those who don't want to help themselves. QUIT worrying about what you've committed to God in prayer. QUIT selling yourself short and settling for less than what God has for you. Friend, you get the picture. Spend today compiling your Quit List in order to make your life better.

My prayer for today is:

_____

_____

_____

What I will do today to embrace this season in my life:

_____

_____

_____

_____

My thoughts for today:

_____

_____

_____

_____

_____

September 7th

Thought of the Day

You can't complain about who and what YOU give power to that affects your life. It's YOUR mind. It's YOUR heart. It's YOUR spirit. It's your TIME. It's YOUR space. It's YOUR money. They're YOUR emotions. Ultimately, it's YOUR discernment and decision that determines who and what has no access, limited access, or all access to the fabric of your being. Be wise and protect your most important asset—YOU.

My prayer for today is:

_____

_____

_____

What I will do today to embrace this season in my life:

_____

_____

_____

_____

My thoughts for today:

_____

_____

_____

_____

September 8th

Thought of the Day

At some point, the focus has to shift from what you're going through to how you are going to get through it. There's too much worth in your life to keep wallowing and worrying in pain and pity. Get up. Get started on your way. Enjoy newness. Let yesterday be a building block for your future.

My prayer for today is:

_____

_____

_____

What I will do today to embrace this season in my life:

_____

_____

_____

_____

My thoughts for today:

_____

_____

_____

_____

September 9th

Thought of the Day

As we mature, many people get to the point where they value peace more than power. They've learned the art of letting stuff go. To do so often allows your mind, your spirit, your attitude, and even your relationships to be free.

My prayer for today is:

_____

_____

_____

What I will do today to embrace this season in my life:

_____

_____

_____

_____

My thoughts for today:

_____

_____

_____

_____

_____

September 10th

Thought of the Day

The real you is never manufactured. It's manifested. In other words, you never have to try to be yourself. Instead, the personality, demeanor, attitude, and approach to various situations shines through no matter where you are, who is around, or what others say or do. Always let the real you shine forth. That's because it takes too much effort to keep up a facade. At the end of the day, you have to go home and look at the real you in the mirror anyway.

My prayer for today is:

_____

_____

_____

What I will do today to embrace this season in my life:

_____

_____

_____

_____

My thoughts for today:

_____

_____

_____

_____

September 11th

Thought of the Day

The old sports adage holds true for life: you win some, you lose some. Just make sure that life's victories are celebrated with humility, gratefulness, and graciousness. View life's defeats as valuable lessons that you'll use to make you better. After the loss, get up and try again. Life is not a one-game, winner-take-all thing. Life is a series full of wins and losses, ups and downs. The key is keep playing, because you're a champion and you're bound for the winner's circle.

My prayer for today is:

_____

_____

_____

What I will do today to embrace this season in my life:

_____

_____

_____

_____

My thoughts for today:

_____

_____

_____

_____

September 12th

Thought of the Day

Life will occasionally place us at four-way crossroads. We can opt to 1) do things our way, 2) do things to please others, 3) do nothing at all, or 4) do things God's way. Friend, there is no argument here. There is nothing to ponder. There should be no conflict at all. To do things God's way is to see the goodness of the Lord on and in your life. It's also to live in peace and not eventually in pieces mentally, emotionally, and spiritually. Let's go all out and follow God's way.

My prayer for today is:

_____

_____

_____

What I will do today to embrace this season in my life:

_____

_____

_____

My thoughts for today:

_____

_____

_____

_____

September 13th

Thought of the Day

One of the things I find exciting in football is when the runner has the ball and is dashing toward the end zone. He's on his way, but a big, 300-pound guy ahead is waiting to tackle him and bring him down. Out of nowhere come's the runner's teammate to block for him. His teammate runs into the would-be tackler and bulldozes him down so that the runner has a clear path to the end zone. How can this apply to your life? Be assured that there is not one thing, neither is there any person, with the ability to stop or block what God intends to do in your life and for your life. Focus on God and watch Him be faithful to you regardless of what others say or do. It is true that if God is with us it's more than the whole world against us. Watch Him take away your tacklers and clear your path!

My prayer for today is:

_____

_____

_____

What I will do today to embrace this season in my life:

_____

_____

_____

_____

My thoughts for today:

_____

_____

_____

_____

_____

September 14th

Thought of the Day

Your outlook on life, certain situations, and even other people largely depend on what's going on deep within you. A thorough self-exam often will bring clarity and focus on everything else. Look in before you look out. Get help if you can't get it together by yourself. There's no shame in making sure you're at the top of your game! Now, have a focused day!

My prayer for today is:

_____

_____

_____

What I will do today to embrace this season in my life:

_____

_____

_____

My thoughts for today:

_____

_____

_____

_____

September 15th

Thought of the Day

God is willing to work on your behalf. But first YOU must be willing to work on your behalf. Put in the prayer, planning, processes, and productivity. Do your absolute best. Then watch God do the rest. There is no need for the SUPERnatural when you haven't done all you can in the NATURAL. Do your thing!

My prayer for today is:

_____

_____

_____

What I will do today to embrace this season in my life:

_____

_____

_____

_____

My thoughts for today:

_____

_____

_____

_____

_____

September 16th

Thought of the Day

The reality is things can't change AROUND you if change doesn't begin WITHIN you. Often a simple change in attitude, mindset, and subsequently determination is all that's needed to set in motion actions and decisions that will lead you to success beyond even what you've dreamed about.

My prayer for today is:

_____

_____

_____

What I will do today to embrace this season in my life:

_____

_____

_____

_____

My thoughts for today:

_____

_____

_____

_____

_____

September 17th

Thought of the Day

A coach and his team worked hard in practice an entire week for a big game. Early in the game, the team got behind by a huge margin. The coach called a timeout and told his players, "Guys, we're behind. Don't worry. Keep believing in what we believe and keep doing what we do and we'll come out on top." The players listened and won the game. That's your word, my friend. Times will come when it seems the enemy is beating the brakes off of you. But keep believing what you believe--that God cares, God is capable, and God will step in right in the nick of time. Then keep doing what you do--praise God, worship God, have integrity, and help others. Eventually, things will turn in your favor and you will be victorious! Fight on. You were born to win!

My prayer for today is:

_____

_____

_____

What I will do today to embrace this season in my life:

_____

_____

_____

_____

My thoughts for today:

_____

_____

_____

_____

_____

September 18th

Thought of the Day

The energy you use to complain can be redirected to find and execute a solution to the complaint. Don't be a sulker—be a solver. How often have we told someone when they asked how we're doing, "I can't complain. It wouldn't help if I did." Or, "I can't complain. No one would care if I did." These are both common quips but they couldn't be more true! Don't spend your time complaining. Aim toward a solution.

My prayer for today is:

_____

_____

_____

What I will do today to embrace this season in my life:

_____

_____

_____

My thoughts for today:

_____

_____

_____

_____

September 19th

Thought of the Day

Though our battles belong to the Lord, we still have to show up, be competent, be confident, be courageous, be determined, be disciplined, be zealous, and be full of faith in order to be the beneficiary of the Lord's blessings. Make it a victorious day!

My prayer for today is:

_____

_____

_____

What I will do today to embrace this season in my life:

_____

_____

_____

_____

My thoughts for today:

_____

_____

_____

_____

_____

September 20th

Thought of the Day

Simple thought. What's too hard for you is always just right for God. There is NOTHING our God can't handle. Put every issue, concern, and situation in His hands and watch Him do exactly what needs to be done. Now, WALK IT OUT IN FAITH on this FAITH-FILLED day!

My prayer for today is:

_____

_____

_____

What I will do today to embrace this season in my life:

_____

_____

_____

_____

My thoughts for today:

_____

_____

_____

_____

_____

September 21st

Thought of the Day

So what if others doubt you! You don't move by their opinions, and God is not moved by their opinions. You and God have the final say over your life. Defeat doubters by expecting greater things and then by executing and excelling. Walk in favor!

My prayer for today is:

_____

_____

_____

What I will do today to embrace this season in my life:

_____

_____

_____

_____

My thoughts for today:

_____

_____

_____

_____

_____

September 22nd

Thought of the Day

A stalled car isn't the same as a wrecked one. Fix and correct what made the car stall and then keep it moving. That's your word, my friend. You just had a moment where you stalled. You're not wrecked. A few bumps and dents? Maybe. But there is still a lot of mileage left on your life and a lot of great places life wants to take you. Fix and correct what caused the stall and keep it moving.

My prayer for today is:

_____

_____

_____

What I will do today to embrace this season in my life:

_____

_____

_____

_____

My thoughts for today:

_____

_____

_____

_____

_____

September 23rd

Thought of the Day

You owe no one an apology for being yourself and the blessings you've gotten for doing so. If God made you as unique and original, then you shouldn't waste one second of your life trying to be a duplicate of someone else. Find peace and confidence in who you are!

My prayer for today is:

_____

_____

_____

What I will do today to embrace this season in my life:

_____

_____

_____

_____

My thoughts for today:

_____

_____

_____

_____

_____

September 24th

Thought of the Day

Think about when you turn on red traffic light while driving. The traffic light commands you to stop. However, you can assess your situation and then make a conscious decision that it is safe and beneficial to turn right and keep it moving. There are many times life situations say STOP. Maybe it is crazy co-workers, unexpected circumstances, the negativity of those you trust, or fear that's fighting your faith. Regardless, take a moment and assess the situation, know that God has cleared a way for you to keep progressing, and make the conscious decision to "turn right" according to God's leading and keep it moving. You're on your way to too many great things to just sit still for nothing.

My prayer for today is:

_____

_____

_____

What I will do today to embrace this season in my life:

_____

_____

_____

_____

My thoughts for today:

_____

_____

_____

_____

September 25th

Thought of the Day

Thinking of our Grandmother Rosie this morning, I remember in the summers she'd take apples that had bruises, rotted spots, and even worms in them and use them anyway. She'd simply cut out the bad spots and make great use of what was left over of the apples for preserves, pies, and just some good ole' stewed apples. God does us the same way. He could've gotten rid of us and our issues a long time ago. Instead, He decided to "cut out" and forgive all of our "bad spots" and use what was "left over" in our lives for His glory. Praise God today that He specializes in using leftovers!

My prayer for today is:

_____

_____

_____

What I will do today to embrace this season in my life:

_____

_____

_____

_____

My thoughts for today:

_____

_____

_____

_____

_____

September 26th

Thought of the Day

Most often your character, integrity, what you stand for, and WHO you stand for (our Father) need not be addressed, defended, or justified. Critics are just that—critics. You can't guide their thoughts or words. However, it's prudent that you guard yourself from engaging in their ignorance and insensitivity. Walk it out today by doing two things: BE YOU and DO YOU well!

My prayer for today is:

_____

_____

_____

What I will do today to embrace this season in my life:

_____

_____

_____

_____

My thoughts for today:

_____

_____

_____

_____

_____

September 27th

Thought of the Day

Never seek validation from anyone who didn't give you victory over death, hell, and the grave. In other words, victory is only in Jesus. Therefore, please Him and gain peace from Him while you watch Him protect you and provide for you. He'll also carry you and care for you through whatever circumstance you may face.

My prayer for today is:

_____

_____

_____

What I will do today to embrace this season in my life:

_____

_____

_____

_____

My thoughts for today:

_____

_____

_____

_____

_____

September 28th

Thought of the Day

It's perfectly okay not to be perfect. Just know that God did not make a mistake when He made you. Therefore, just be you. Then know it's okay to "do you." Most of all, resolve that you will allow God to continually mold and shape every aspect of your life to be just as He desires. Be okay with who you are, but know that you're by no means a finished product. You can still shape the world while you're being shaped.

My prayer for today is:

_____

_____

_____

What I will do today to embrace this season in my life:

_____

_____

_____

_____

My thoughts for today:

_____

_____

_____

_____

September 29th

Thought of the Day

Remember that sometimes it's only in your greatest challenges that you realize just how strong you really are. Adversity is not so much to "punish" you as Satan would have you to believe. Often God uses our adversities to "prove" the confidence, determination, focus, grit, and power that He has put within you.

My prayer for today is:

_____

_____

_____

What I will do today to embrace this season in my life:

_____

_____

_____

_____

My thoughts for today:

_____

_____

_____

_____

September 30th

Thought of the Day

You woke up. You have sight. You have a roof over your head. Your legs and arms move. You have your right mind. You have food. You have clothing. Friend, it's already been a mighty good day for you. Yes, each day brings challenges and at times frustrations. However, never let your mind stall on those things. Instead, focus on the blessings and remember that the same God who blessed you to see the day is the same God who will see you through the day.

My prayer for today is:

_____

_____

_____

What I will do today to embrace this season in my life:

_____

_____

_____

_____

My thoughts for today:

_____

_____

_____

_____

_____

October

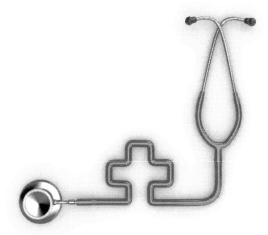

October
Trick or Treat

Medicine

October 31st is observed in various ways. We are all familiar with kids in costumes ringing doorbells saying, "Trick or treat." Many churches choose to have family-friendly trunk or treat. Even though there can be some negative interpretations of that date, I think most of us have found ways to make it a family-friendly time for socialization. We find ways for kids to be kids as we adults reminisce on what it was like to be their age. Even the candy in the stores brings back fond memories as we eye some of our all-time favorites from when we were children. My son laughs when I want to buy a bag that has Baby Ruth miniatures and individual-size boxes of Milk Duds. He says the children will rebel at my "old-school candy." What? That is the stuff sweet dreams are made of! And yes, I do eat sweets—in moderation!

As much as I like my old-school candy for the taste, I love the memories. I remember watching *It's the Great Pumpkin Charlie Brown* with Papa while he pretended he hated the candy we loved. This alleged hatred of our snacks would compel him to pop popcorn for us to enjoy together. After smiling at that memory, I move on down the grocery store aisle with my son to buy cute little bags of pretzels with festive designs to give kids. My son then asks if I want kids to hate us! I can't win with him. I buy them anyway for kids who shouldn't ingest lots of sugar from candy. We keep walking through the store watching as kids marvel at different costumes and masks. It's all fun to them.

Seriousness does come to mind. I think the reason some people enjoy wearing masks—whether on October 31st or other occasions such as a masquerade ball—is that, for a short time, they get to be someone or something else. The mask can hide the real expressions they wear on their faces. Too often, we also wear masks in our daily lives. We think as long as we smile, no one can see what we're really struggling with. We may pretend we're happily toasting at a gathering with a cocktail when we're really trying to numb our sorrows. We have to stop tricking ourselves that way. Everyone has good days and bad days. However, if there are more bad days than good days, we may need help to get balance back into our lives. We may find the best treats of our lives through the process.

Why are we hesitant to seek help? When we think of some of the psalms, David directly petitioned God in his anguish and God delivered him. We want that to be our story as well. And sometimes, it may be. We all go through peaks and valleys. The problem is when we dwell in the valley. There are other stories in the Bible such as the one that surrounds Nebuchadnezzar's dream in Daniel 2. The king was troubled and could not sleep. He summoned astrologers and wise men to interpret his dream. Daniel, a man of God, gave the king counsel by interpreting his dream. Daniel was clear that his gift came from God.

My point is that God works in different ways. The Bible says that God is not the author of confusion. Right, preacher?

Ministry

You're referring to 1 Corinthians 14 when Paul addressed confusion and strife in the church. He relayed the fact that confusion in the church doesn't come from God. And while Paul was talking specifically about the body of Christ, I think it not robbery to make the statement applicable to our relationships and even our minds. God wants our minds, hearts, and spirits free. The last thing He wants is anxiety and confusion deep within us. That's the desire and ultimately the plan of Satan. Stability of the saints is a direct enemy of Satan! The last thing he wants is for believers to have a clear, focused mind. That's why Paul called for us to be transformed by having our mind renewed by the Holy Spirit daily—actually several times daily.

There is value in a free, faith-filled, and focused mind. This is true from both spiritual health and mental health aspects. That's why in both areas there is immense value in seeking counsel, advice, and therapy from qualified spiritual counselors, licensed counselors, and/or mental health professionals. God places people in our paths often for the sole purpose of keeping us on the right path. Or, in some instances, we all need a little help at times getting back on the right path.

It's important for believers to know that you're not weak because you seek help. You aren't some spiritual infidel because your personal prayer time and devotion aren't enough to get you to the mental and spiritual space you desire. You're not fake or hypocritical to minister to others and yet need ministering to yourself. Even the most expensive car needs servicing every now and then. Our smartphones need recharging and an occasional reset. It's the same with the saints. Sometimes we need to seek help in order to get a needed spiritual, mental, emotional, and physical *tune-up*. If you don't seek help, will you keep living? Sure. However, like a car that needs a tune-up, you'll function, but not optimally and smoothly.

October

Our prayer for you this month is that you don't hide behind any mask and that you love your authentic self. What are your goals for this month?

1.

2

3.

October 1st

Thought of the Day

So many people wear crosses around their necks. The way they carry themselves determines if the crosses are just pieces of jewelry or symbols of faith. Is your cross just bling or does it show you are a child of the King?

My prayer for today is:

_____

_____

_____

What I will do today to be my authentic self:

_____

_____

_____

_____

My thoughts for today:

_____

_____

_____

_____

_____

October 2nd

Thought of the Day

We often try to pacify ourselves with comfort food, alcohol, or drugs. The problem is that these things never actually fill the void. By the time we realize that, we're so much further away from where we want to be. Make up your mind that you will turn your situation around by addressing the root of your problem. U-turns are allowed on the streets of life.

My prayer for today is:

_____

_____

_____

What I will do today to be my authentic self:

_____

_____

_____

My thoughts for today:

_____

_____

_____

_____

October 3rd

Thought of the Day

Author Kim Culbertson has a great saying, "People think being alone makes you lonely, but I don't think that's true. Being surrounded by the wrong people is the loneliest thing in the world." I bet most of us know that from our own experiences. The goal is never to be in a crowd that forgets you're there and can trample you if trouble breaks out. I'd rather be a part of a circle that holds its shape because of the well-rounded people in it. If trouble breaks out in my circle, my friends hold me up while I'm also making sure they don't fall.

My prayer for today is:

_____

_____

_____

What I will do today to be my authentic self:

_____

_____

_____

_____

My thoughts for today:

_____

_____

_____

_____

_____

October 4ᵗʰ

Thought of the Day

One of my favorite Bible verses is Galatians 6:9 (KJV): "And let us not be weary in well doing; for in due season we shall reap, if we faint not." For me, that translates into motivation to keep fighting the good fight. That can be applied to so many things, including fighting for your health and wellness. It will ultimately pay off. Keep going. You got this!

My prayer for today is:

_____

_____

_____

What I will do today to be my authentic self:

_____

_____

_____

My thoughts for today:

_____

_____

_____

_____

October 5th

Thought of the Day

Don't pretend you are good with the way things are in your life because you are overwhelmed at the thought of what you have to do to make them better. Some people seem to have it all together, and we quickly want to proclaim that it just isn't fair. We don't see the work that they put in to keep it together. The sooner we get past the notion that there is a quick fix for sustained gains, the quicker we can move on to embracing the needed changes in our lives.

My prayer for today is:

_____

_____

_____

What I will do today to be my authentic self:

_____

_____

_____

_____

My thoughts for today:

_____

_____

_____

_____

October 6th

Thought of the Day

Sometimes people say interesting things when they don't want to give up their vices. They may say, "I got to die of something." The sad thing is that if they do die of something preventable, they are gone, but their loved ones are left to keep reliving what could have been. Live to truly live. Don't live to die. It affects more than you.

My prayer for today is:

_____

_____

_____

What I will do today to be my authentic self:

_____

_____

_____

_____

My thoughts for today:

_____

_____

_____

_____

October 7th

Thought of the Day

We really can't "lose" our focus. That's because we choose what people, what things, what places, and what situations to focus on. Therefore, our focus is never lost; but it's always given. Make a conscious decision to carefully choose your focal points on this BLESSED day.

My prayer for today is:

_____

_____

_____

What I will do today to be my authentic self:

_____

_____

_____

_____

My thoughts for today:

_____

_____

_____

_____

_____

October 8th

Thought of the Day

Sometimes life will produce some unforeseen, unplanned, and unfortunate detours and distractions. Never let them unravel your plans and unhinge your faith. Your goals are still intact. Your destiny and ultimate destination are still valid and ahead. Take a breath. Then take your time and navigate the detours. Be determined never to stop. Before you know it, you'll arrive exactly where God wants you to be at the time God wants you to be there.

My prayer for today is:

_____

_____

_____

What I will do today to be my authentic self:

_____

_____

_____

_____

My thoughts for today:

_____

_____

_____

_____

_____

October 9th

Thought of the Day

No matter what others think or say, how you treat people and the way you live in front of people daily are the two things that truly write the script of your life. This life script will stand despite how much hype or how much hell someone else gives you. This life script establishes your name regardless of what's being expressed about your name. Live each day knowing that your life—your words, actions, attitude, and disposition—tells the whole story!

My prayer for today is:

_____

_____

_____

What I will do today to be my authentic self:

_____

_____

_____

My thoughts for today:

_____

_____

_____

_____

October 10th

Thought of the Day

Doubt and fear are distracting, disruptive, and destructive devices of the enemy to keep your eyes from seeing your goals and the rewards that accompany them, to keep your mind from thinking that the "best you" hasn't been unveiled yet, and to keep your heart from believing that there is nothing you can't do with the power and help of God. Defeat doubts and fears with words of faith. Once your faith is firmly in place, the subsequent work needed to bring hopes, dreams, goals, and your best to reality will follow.

My prayer for today is:

_____

_____

_____

What I will do today to be my authentic self:

_____

_____

_____

_____

My thoughts for today:

_____

_____

_____

_____

_____

October 11th

Thought of the Day

Believe in yourself enough and be so motivated that you refuse to quit or even slow down until your hopes and your dreams become reality! This is all about you and God and no one else! Be good with that and make the very best of your opportunities. Now, walk it out!

My prayer for today is:

_____

_____

_____

What I will do today to be my authentic self:

_____

_____

_____

_____

My thoughts for today:

_____

_____

_____

_____

_____

October 12th

Thought of the Day

You don't need everyone to understand you and your every move as long as YOU understand that God is working IN you and THROUGH you for His glory! Your best is yet to come because God has yet to reveal and release all He has planned for your life. Keep pressing and believing!

My prayer for today is:

_____

_____

_____

What I will do today to be my authentic self:

_____

_____

_____

_____

My thoughts for today:

_____

_____

_____

_____

_____

October 13th

Thought of the Day

Worry is a spiritual enemy of an active and effective prayer life. If you're going to worry, doubt will creep in and there's not much need to pray. If you're going to pray in faith, doubts should be defeated and worry should be abated. So which will drive you—worry or faith? Choose faith!

My prayer for today is:

_____

_____

_____

What I will do today to be my authentic self:

_____

_____

_____

_____

My thoughts for today:

_____

_____

_____

_____

_____

October 14th

Thought of the Day

Don't miss taking advantage of open doors trying to rationalize with people who have closed minds. Their opinions will only provide obstacles that have the ability to cause you to squander favor and opportunities. Keep going forward in your faith.

My prayer for today is:

_____

_____

_____

What I will do today to be my authentic self:

_____

_____

_____

_____

My thoughts for today:

_____

_____

_____

_____

October 15th

Thought of the Day

My maternal grandfather would always say, "Speak to everyone. Your car could be broken down by the side of the road. If people remember you from your kindness, they will be more likely to stop." Here's a couple of questions for you. Would someone you met in passing be willing to come to your aid? If that same someone needed help, would they be glad to see you coming? Don't let your demeanor make those answers be "no."

My prayer for today is:

_____

_____

_____

What I will do today to be my authentic self:

_____

_____

_____

_____

My thoughts for today:

_____

_____

_____

_____

_____

October 16th

Thought of the Day

Friend, today I want to encourage you to GIVE UP! Yes, you need to GIVE UP! Give up worrying; trust God is working it out. Give up trying to please everybody; make sure God is pleased. Give up being so hard on yourself; God wants you to move on. Give up feeling you're not worth it; God sent Jesus to die for you. So, He obviously thinks otherwise. Give up fear; faith looks so much better on you. Friend, GIVE UP today. God's got so much in store for you once you GIVE UP the hindrances that keep you from receiving from Him.

My prayer for today is:

_____

_____

_____

What I will do today to be my authentic self:

_____

_____

_____

_____

My thoughts for today:

_____

_____

_____

_____

_____

October 17th

Thought of the Day

Prayer is only effective when your heart believes God will answer the requests that your mouth utters. It's almost like going to the ATM. Most people don't put their cards in the machine if they don't believe they will get something out. That's a transaction based on a relationship. A relationship has been established with the bank ahead of that time. You have set up a process to deposit money. Your expectation is to get your money out when you need it. Likewise, when you have an established relationship with God, you have the confidence to know He will answer your prayers. Don't expect a withdrawal if you never make a deposit.

My prayer for today is:

_____

_____

_____

What I will do today to be my authentic self:

_____

_____

_____

_____

My thoughts for today:

_____

_____

_____

_____

_____

October 18th

Thought of the Day

One day, the power went out at our home for about 10 minutes. The kids went crazy! You'd have thought the world was coming to an end. They couldn't watch their favorite show. Their phones needed charging. It was too dark. The kids were in full crisis mode. I had an opportunity to teach them an important lesson. They did not have a crisis; they had an inconvenience. People without homes have a crisis. The diagnosis some folks just got yesterday presented a crisis. I gave many examples. We had a great talk. Be careful not to label your inconvenience as a crisis. Sometimes a little peek at real darkness helps you to better appreciate the light.

My prayer for today is:

_____

_____

_____

What I will do today to be my authentic self:

_____

_____

_____

_____

My thoughts for today:

_____

_____

_____

_____

_____

October 19th

Thought of the Day

Life really is what we make it to be. If we want to have joy and be joyful, we will. If we want to live in a place of discontent and dissatisfaction, we will. If we want to live healthier, we can. God gives us the canvas called life each day. He puts a brush in our hands each day as well. Ultimately, our minds and hearts will determine what picture we paint.

My prayer for today is:

_____

_____

_____

What I will do today to be my authentic self:

_____

_____

_____

_____

My thoughts for today:

_____

_____

_____

_____

_____

October 20th

Thought of the Day

Sometimes you become a victim because of a situation. Other times, you land in situations because of your victim mentality. You instantly become a victim when you get stuck in sadness for yourself and soreness at everyone else. Life often throws some nasty curveballs that prove hard to hit. Having a victim's mentality causes you to tether yourself to the painful situation. A victor's mentality causes you to label the situation as just temporary. Then you adjust your stance and swing so you can hit that same curveball and make something positive of it. Remember, homeruns are often hit just as the batter was on the brink of a strikeout. Keep swinging for the fences!

My prayer for today is:

_____

_____

_____

What I will do today to be my authentic self:

_____

_____

_____

_____

My thoughts for today:

_____

_____

_____

_____

October 21st

Thought of the Day

The enemy loves to plant seeds of fear into our minds so that we will harvest images of the worst-case scenario for our situation. Operating in fear, we'll keep trying to figure out solutions on our own. Stop a moment. Refocus your faith. Remind yourself that God loves you. Refresh your memory about His power. If He's done it for you before, why wouldn't He do it again? Let your mind be at ease while you wait on God to take care of the situation that you've turned over to Him.

My prayer for today is:

_____

_____

_____

What I will do today to be my authentic self:

_____

_____

_____

_____

My thoughts for today:

_____

_____

_____

_____

_____

October 22nd

Thought of the Day

Often we must wait on God to supply our needs, answer our prayers, open doors, etc. However, a heart full of faith doesn't allow the wait to be weighted with worry! Keep believing while waiting on the blessing!

My prayer for today is:

_____

_____

_____

What I will do today to be my authentic self:

_____

_____

_____

_____

My thoughts for today:

_____

_____

_____

_____

October 23rd

Thought of the Day

We were all trying to live in Wakanda after we saw the movie *Black Panther*. Wakanda had this miraculous substance called vibranium. It was a type of metallic element that held all kinds of energy. It was powerful when used for good. As it is in a superhero movie, it could be devastating if used for evil. Some of the reasons I think we fell in love with Wakanda and its people is that they were powerful but not over-imposing. They were proud but not prideful. They brought people together for good. They fought for noble causes. Wait! Those fictionalized attributes can be practiced in real life. We don't have the gift of vibranium, but we have gifts that can't be taken away that can be used for good. The Bible has all kinds of superheroes. I guess since we are descendants of them, that makes us superheroes, too!

My prayer for today is:

_____

_____

_____

What I will do today to be my authentic self:

_____

_____

_____

_____

My thoughts for today:

_____

_____

_____

_____

_____

October 24th

Thought of the Day

The least of your worries should be explaining yourself and explaining what God is doing in your life to someone who has not invested even a simple, genuine smile or word of encouragement into your life. Stop feeling as is if you owe those people priority and purpose in your life. Why do we concern ourselves over people who don't seem to like us for no apparent reason? Keep being you and know that you aren't responsible for changing their view of you. All you can do is continue to walk in the light.

My prayer for today is:

_____

_____

_____

What I will do today to be my authentic self:

_____

_____

_____

_____

My thoughts for today:

_____

_____

_____

_____

October 25th

Thought of the Day

When your foundation and hope is in Christ, you'll find that you can't and won't be hindered by criticisms from those who have no concept or perception of God's plan and purpose for your life. They can't see what you can nor should they. Your dream and destiny is for you. Keep grinding.

My prayer for today is:

_____

_____

_____

What I will do today to be my authentic self:

_____

_____

_____

My thoughts for today:

_____

_____

_____

_____

October 26th

Thought of the Day

Yesterday, I parked the car and got out with my son. We headed toward the store. As we walked between parked cars, a lady in a car was on her phone laughing when she looked up and saw my son and I walking toward her car as we made our way to the store's front entrance. Instantly, her laugh ceased and a frown and frightened look took over her face. She grabbed her purse, which was on the front seat. I heard the car CLICK! She had locked her doors. At first, it bothered me. But I kept walking calmly and confidently with my son to the store. All I did was be who I'm made to be. These were HER issues, HER insecurities, and HER wayward thoughts—not mine. Friend, you can't control others.

My prayer for today is:

_____

_____

_____

What I will do today to be my authentic self:

_____

_____

_____

_____

My thoughts for today:

_____

_____

_____

_____

October 27th

Thought of the Day

So the enemy, issues, and obstacles seem HUGE to you! Well, remember that was certainly the case when David came face to face with Goliath. But we know how that story ended! All you need is God, faith, and courage and you'll find out that GIANTS DO FALL!

My prayer for today is:

_____

_____

_____

What I will do today to be my authentic self:

_____

_____

_____

_____

My thoughts for today:

_____

_____

_____

_____

_____

October 28th

Thought of the Day

It's one thing to say or think you're strong. It's another thing to KNOW you're strong. Most often the only way to know you're strong is to be tested. Know that many of your tests and trials are not to destroy you but to develop you. Hang in there! You can and will handle what comes your way.

My prayer for today is:

_____

_____

_____

What I will do today to be my authentic self:

_____

_____

_____

My thoughts for today:

_____

_____

_____

_____

October 29th

Thought of the Day

The lines of communication with God are always open. Most often He's just waiting on us to "call" Him through prayer! And when you pray, God desires a dialogue with you. You speak to Him. Then stay "on the line" long enough for Him to speak to your mind, your heart, and your spirit. Phone it in!

My prayer for today is:

_____

_____

_____

What I will do today to be my authentic self:

_____

_____

_____

_____

My thoughts for today:

_____

_____

_____

_____

_____

October 30th

Thought of the Day

Never allow people who don't dare to dream to extinguish the fire and passion you have to chase your hopes and dreams. Don't be mad at them if they want to stay exactly where they are in life. Don't pacify them by staying stagnant with them.

My prayer for today is:

_____

_____

_____

What I will do today to be my authentic self:

_____

_____

_____

_____

My thoughts for today:

_____

_____

_____

_____

_____

October 31ˢᵗ

Thought of the Day

Simple encouragement today—you're alive! So LIVE. You fit neatly into the devil's plans and pleasure when you're consistently stale, stagnant, sore, sorrowful, sad, and scared. God blessed you to be alive another day. So LIVE. Know there is a blessing in your breath.

My prayer for today is:

_____

_____

_____

What I will do today to be my authentic self:

_____

_____

_____

_____

My thoughts for today:

_____

_____

_____

_____

_____

November

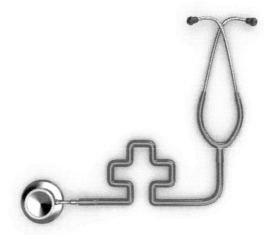

November
Thanksgiving

Medicine

It's probably no surprise to you that the focus for this month is Thanksgiving. You may be surprised that the gist of what I'm going to say is not to skip the big meal with your family or friends. That is such a rich tradition. I think there are good habits we can incorporate like seasoning the greens with smoked turkey versus fattier meats. We can resist going back for that third helping. We know we really shouldn't eat ourselves into comas. We say it's only one day. What can it hurt?

It can hurt because we rarely keep it to one day. Those leftovers tend to call us the next day and, many times, the day after that. Those few holiday pounds get harder and harder to shed each year. Thanksgiving is another one of those times that my trainer says eat what you want but you will pay for it. He is signaling that the post-Thanksgiving workouts with the new acquired abdominal girth will be a reminder that if you play, you pay. Even though I am mad at him during the workouts, I get it. It's not about trying to be perfect. It is about taking personal responsibility for your health.

Sadly, sometimes we don't want to get healthy or stay healthy for ourselves. But if you look around the Thanksgiving table, I bet there are people sitting there who you want to be around for. It may be that spouse who has been your rock who needs you now more than ever. It may be those grandkids you want to see grow up. It may be that best friend you love like a sibling who is dreaming up vacation plans that include you. If it's not a person, maybe it's your lifelong dreams that could be your compelling reason to stay healthy. Sometimes we have become blinded to the good reasons to be around even when they are right before our eyes.

I mentioned I have run half marathons. I usually try to pick races that support a charity I believe in. That motivates me. During my very first half marathon that I trained so poorly for, I was struggling and questioned if I would complete it. I told myself I could not do it. I came across a group of young amputees cheering us runners on. They were so happy and genuine in their support. Before I knew it, tears streaked down my cheeks. I told myself that I could no longer say, "I can't run." There were these cheering children who couldn't run and still had joy. I may not always want to run, but I had limbs that worked. I could run. I have never forgotten that.

I dragged my son into running kicking and screaming. I told him we had to run for those who can't run for themselves. There are many runs for charity on Thanksgiving morning. My son and I did an 8K Thanksgiving morning benefitting those with chronic kidney disease. Later that day, we joined our family for a wonderful dinner. My point is this. Thanksgiving can include new traditions. If you don't run, you can walk. These races not only give to good causes, but they give the participants even more reasons to count their blessings. I run for those who can't run for themselves, believing that should a day come that I can't run for myself, someone will have the heart to run for me. Psalm 100:4 says to enter His gates with thanksgiving. I'm pretty sure God won't mind me entering with running shoes on, will He, preacher?

Ministry

No. I'm sure He's cool with us coming in with running shoes. The fact is, we can still be very active during the holiday season. Just truly caring and sharing can give us needed exercise. I pastor the New Life Church in Athens, Alabama. I'm proud to say that we love to share the love of Christ during the holidays—and all year round. While doing so, we also get some exercise in.

Each year, we sponsor what we proudly call The King's Table Community Thanksgiving Meal. On a Saturday in early November, we invite the community to come to our campus for a free, delicious Thanksgiving meal. We literally feed hundreds of people each year. Preparation, execution, and post-event activities are very labor-intensive. We stack chairs, set tables, and serve tables. Then we break down tables, replace chairs, etc. We even take hundreds of plates to local hotels where transients stay to ensure anyone who wants food gets it. It's a great ministry opportunity that blesses people and glorifies God. However, it also provides so much needed cardio, lifting, walking, and other key exercises.

During the holidays, be active. Volunteer at church. Serve in a soup kitchen. Don't just sit around, eat, and be miserable. Enjoy the season but also find ways to use the season to get in a few needed reps of exercise.

November

Our prayer for you this month is really simple. We pray that you don't treat Thanksgiving as just one day to give thanks. Our hope is that thanksgiving is your posture the entire month and even the entire year. What are your goals for this month?

1.

2.

3.

November 1st

Thought of the Day:

I truly believe that there are some blessings that God has for us that are in layaway until we develop a true heart of gratitude, thank Him, and openly praise Him for all He's already done for us and through us. It really shouldn't be that hard. One of the reasons He created us is so that we will forever worship, praise, and magnify Him. Friend, give God what He deserves on this MARVELOUS day!

My prayer for today is:

_____

_____

_____

What I am thankful for today:

_____

_____

_____

My thoughts for today:

_____

_____

_____

_____

November 2nd

Thought of the Day

You don't have to be "deep" to find a reason to be grateful. Watch television for 10 minutes and you'll find that, unfortunately, these days simply making it home from the store is a very valid reason to give God thanks. Thank the Lord for all He's done. All of my life I've heard the seasoned saints of the church sing the ageless song, *I'm Satisfied With Jesus*. I woke up this morning with that song ringing in my heart, mind, and spirit. However, one verse hit a little differently today than it ever has before. I can hear some of the older saints with a passionate plea in song saying, "You can't make me doubt Him in my heart. Because I know too much about Him." Don't ask me why that one verse blessed me tremendously today! But it did. I hope it makes you think about your experiences, your faith, and God's faithfulness to you today also!

My prayer for today is:

_____

_____

_____

What I am thankful for today:

_____

_____

_____

_____

My thoughts for today:

_____

_____

_____

_____

November 3rd

Thought of the Day

Can't seem to find much to be thankful about? Try this. Take a deep breath. Put your hand in front of your mouth. Exhale. Did you feel your breath coming from your body? Yes? This one thing is enough for you to praise God all day long. Life in and of itself is a blessing that ought not ever be taken for granted. Give Him praise on this thankful day.

My prayer for today is:

_____

_____

_____

What I am thankful for today:

_____

_____

_____

_____

My thoughts for today:

_____

_____

_____

_____

_____

November 4th

Thought of the Day

Three words for you today, my friend JUST BE GRATEFUL! Things may not be as well as you'd like them to be. However, they certainly can be worse than they are right now. Some among us would consider what we call "a problem" as a blessing. Spend today thinking of the goodness of God and then tell Him, "Father, I'm grateful for all you've done, all you're doing, and all you will do in my life."

My prayer for today is:

_____

_____

_____

What I am thankful for today:

_____

_____

_____

My thoughts for today:

_____

_____

_____

_____

_____

November 5th

Thought of the Day

My son and I had the opportunity to visit the famous leaning tower of Pisa. We entered the tower with a group. We were so happy to be at the lead of our group because we could easily jog up the stairs. We didn't realize that the stairs start on the inside of the tower and near the top are on the outside of the wall. You should have seen us when we hit the outside. We were so high up that we absolutely froze in fear. Our group caught up to us, and we still could not move. We were petrified. As a mother, I knew that I needed to comfort and guide my son out of the situation. As I slowly thawed from my fear, a couple from England right behind us told us everything was going to be alright and that we could hold on to them if we needed to. We saw God in that moment. We were able to get to the top where we stood next to a blind man and his guide who had successfully navigated the stairs. The blind man asked his guide to describe the view from the top as the wind gently blew on his face. We listened. The guide was eloquent, and it was clear the blind man was picturing the scene as vividly as if he had sight. We realized that we took our blessings for granted. We gratefully stood at the top as we saw Pisa with our own eyes as well as through the blind man's eyes.

My prayer for today is:

_____

_____

_____

What I am thankful for today:

_____

_____

_____

_____

My thoughts for today:

_____

_____

_____

_____

_____

November 6th

Thought of the Day

We must learn that at times victory and strength are in silence. Everything need not get a response. Everyone need not be addressed. The discipline of silence will often defeat your enemies and derail your enemy's plans against you. Learn that silence is not weakness. Often, it's the evidence of strength laced in wisdom.

My prayer for today is:

_____

_____

_____

What I am thankful for today:

_____

_____

_____

_____

My thoughts for today:

_____

_____

_____

_____

_____

November 7th

Thought of the Day

I made sweet potato pies for Thanksgiving one year. My son nearly ate a whole one by himself. He got sick. To this day, he won't eat sweet potato pie. I remind him that he actually loved the pie. The pie didn't make him sick, his overindulgence made him sick. Sometimes it's like that in life as well. We'll point to something else being the problem, and we can't admit that it's really our behavior that's the problem. We ask ourselves questions like, Why do I keep attracting the wrong mate? Why do I keep ending up at the wrong job? Why can't I keep my weight off when I strictly follow the fad diets? If you have a consistent string of wrongs, look in the mirror at the person who holds the power to get it right.

My prayer for today is:

_____

_____

_____

What I am thankful for today:

_____

_____

_____

My thoughts for today:

_____

_____

_____

_____

November 8th

Thought of the Day

A very simple way to handle difficult times in your life is to declare to yourself, "It is what it is. But it isn't what it's going to be." By faith, believe that sooner or later things really are going to turn in your favor. Keep your head up!

My prayer for today is:

_____

_____

_____

What I am thankful for today:

_____

_____

_____

_____

My thoughts for today:

_____

_____

_____

_____

_____

November 9th

Thought of the Day

If you're saved and growing in God, there is one thing we should immensely, intentionally, and continually praise God for. We should praise Him that who we are now doesn't resemble who we used to be. Praise Him that you don't walk, talk, and live the way you used to. Why? Because HE made the difference! Show Him gratitude by showing others your makeover.

My prayer for today is:

_____

_____

_____

What I am thankful for today:

_____

_____

_____

_____

My thoughts for today:

_____

_____

_____

_____

_____

November 10th

Thought of the Day

Never get it twisted. We can't and don't "impress" God with anything we have, anything we do, anything we say, or any title or accolade we possess. He's not moved by any of these things. However, He IS moved by our love for Him and others, our commitment to kingdom matters, our prayer life that seeks to dialogue with Him, and our worship that simply adores Him for who He is. Those who grasp this truth understand life is not about impressing but pleasing the one who matters most--our God!

My prayer for today is:

_____

_____

_____

What I am thankful for today:

_____

_____

_____

_____

My thoughts for today:

_____

_____

_____

_____

_____

November 11th

Thought of the Day

Seven words to strengthen your resolve to never quit, to keep the faith, and to keep pressing forward — God is able and He won't fail. Think on these words today, my friend. By faith, they'll make a world of difference in your current situation. You can even repeat these words as you're going for that walk or run. It's nothing like moving to a mantra that matters!

My prayer for today is:

_____

_____

_____

What I am thankful for today:

_____

_____

_____

_____

My thoughts for today:

_____

_____

_____

_____

_____

November 12th

Thought of the Day

When I drive, I am very conscious about thanking people when they're courteous enough to allow me to switch lanes in front of them. The very least I can do is look back in my rear-view mirror, see who's done something good for me, and wave my hand in gratitude. That's your word, my friend. When you look back over your life and see just how good God has been and how much He's done for you, wave your hand with an attitude of gratitude. God's graciousness is often invoked by our gratefulness. Be grateful!

My prayer for today is:

_____

_____

_____

What I am thankful for today:

_____

_____

_____

_____

My thoughts for today:

_____

_____

_____

_____

November 13th

Thought of the Day

Our daughter, Emani, and I washed my wife's car recently. As Emani played with the water, she shouted "Daddy, we need to call the water people because the water doesn't work anymore!" In actuality, there was a kink in the hose. I explained to her that "the water people" were still doing their job by supplying all the water we needed; but it was our responsibility to get rid of kinks. Friend, God is doing His job by supplying all you need and much of what you want. It's your job to identify the "kinks"—the people, actions, mindsets, and such that are blocking your blessings! Undo the kinks and watch the blessings flow into your life!

My prayer for today is:

What I am thankful for today:

My thoughts for today:

November 14th

Thought of the Day

In life's toughest times, focus on God's ability rather than your inability. Be calmed and comforted by two words today: He's able! When you know that you know that He's able, you will also know you are capable! Go forth in confidence!

My prayer for today is:

_____

_____

_____

What I am thankful for today:

_____

_____

_____

_____

My thoughts for today:

_____

_____

_____

_____

_____

November 15th

Thought of the Day

Complaining is a great strategy of the enemy. It does two things. It clouds your concentration of just how good God is, and it contaminates the attitudes and spirits of those around you. Spend today counting your blessings rather than complaining.

My prayer for today is:

_____

_____

_____

What I am thankful for today:

_____

_____

_____

_____

My thoughts for today:

_____

_____

_____

_____

November 16th

Thought of the Day

Remember that God is never slow concerning us and our needs. Instead, we often are impatient concerning His will, His way, and His timing. God knows what's best for us even if it doesn't match our timelines or deadlines. Remember, God is faithful.

My prayer for today is:

_____

_____

_____

What I am thankful for today:

_____

_____

_____

My thoughts for today:

_____

_____

_____

_____

November 17th

Thought of the Day

We should never stop praising God. After all, He never stops providing for us. He NEVER stops protecting us. He NEVER stops giving us peace when we need it most. He NEVER stops giving us power to endure rough times. To this point, He has NEVER stopped waking us up. Furthermore, He KEEPS ON blessings us over and over again. Therefore, from the rising of the sun to the going down of the same, we should PRAISE God for all He's done, all He's doing, and all He's going to do.

My prayer for today is:

_____

_____

_____

What I am thankful for today:

_____

_____

_____

_____

My thoughts for today:

_____

_____

_____

_____

November 18th

Thought of the Day

How many times have you driven places with absolutely no clue where you were going? Chances are you didn't worry at all as long as you had your navigation device on and talking. Life is very similar. There will be times that God doesn't reveal every step and turn you'll take. Still, "drive on" like you do with your navigator. And don't worry! Like the navigator, God is with you all the way. Unlike the navigator, God is ALREADY in the very place He's taking you. Trust Him as He orders your steps and makes plain your path.

My prayer for today is:

_____

_____

_____

What I am thankful for today:

_____

_____

_____

_____

My thoughts for today:

_____

_____

_____

_____

_____

November 19th

Thought of the Day

FACT: You're reading this passage. FACT: That means you're alive. FACT: God looked past your faults, flaws, and failures and blessed you with another day and another chance. FACT: You should thank Him right now for HIS grace and mercy toward you. FACT: He is worthy of our praise. You know where you can dwell on these facts—on your walk or your run today. Just saying…!

My prayer for today is:

_____

_____

_____

What I am thankful for today:

_____

_____

_____

_____

My thoughts for today:

_____

_____

_____

_____

November 20th

Thought of the Day

The word for today is "patience." Know that patience simply "presses pause" on life's moments at times. However, patience never forfeits life's missions and ministries. There is a huge difference between being delayed and being derailed. Keep working with focus and faithfulness. You're still on the tracks, so keep moving forward.

My prayer for today is:

_____

_____

_____

What I am thankful for today:

_____

_____

_____

_____

My thoughts for today:

_____

_____

_____

_____

November 21st

Thought of the Day

Friend, we follow our focus! That means our actions and affections are most often given to the things and people that grab and hold our attention. It's on you today to focus positively and passionately so that you can be progressive and productive in all that you endeavor. Make the most of this marvelous day.

My prayer for today is:

_____

_____

_____

What I am thankful for today:

_____

_____

_____

_____

My thoughts for today:

_____

_____

_____

_____

_____

November 22nd

Thought of the Day

Some of the nicest chapels are in hospitals. Why is that? If a loved one is having a long surgery, all we can do is wait. Sometimes we just wait in the waiting room or we may visit the chapel. In those moments, we realize that all we can do is wait. We petition God to guide the surgeon's hands. We ask that God be with our loved one. We ask God to be with us and to calm our fears. While these situations are tense, recognize that God is omnipotent. Believe the Lord will answer your prayers and act on your behalf. When the answer you have been waiting for manifests, don't forget to thank God. And don't make Him wait until your next crisis to hear from you again.

My prayer for today is:

_____

_____

_____

What I am thankful for today:

_____

_____

_____

_____

My thoughts for today:

_____

_____

_____

_____

November 23rd

Thought of the Day

I've said before I feel the fitness journey can parallel the Christian journey. Here's an example. Sometimes the scale can be deceptive. You watch your numbers fall, fall, fall, and then, out of nowhere, you gain 2 pounds! You didn't do anything differently. You exercised, you ate right, you drank your water, and you got sleep. It happens! Don't deem your journey a lost cause! In life and fitness, don't let a temporary setback keep you from your long-term goal. Push through it. Sometimes progress pauses but it IS still progress. You might have to change your path. The important part is that you get to your destination.

My prayer for today is:

_____

_____

_____

What I am thankful for today:

_____

_____

_____

My thoughts for today:

_____

_____

_____

_____

November 24th

Thought of the Day

Christmas decorations go on display right after the Halloween costumes are packed up in the stores. Thanksgiving doesn't seem to get much of the highlight at all. There are a few decorations that say "blessings" or "Thanksgiving." I bought some Thanksgiving glassware last year that say, "Grateful Hearts" and "Count Your Blessings." I love those glasses. I use them year-round because they reflect how I feel. The reality is that we don't need retail to help us celebrate what should be in our hearts all year.

My prayer for today is:

_____

_____

_____

What I am thankful for today:

_____

_____

_____

_____

My thoughts for today:

_____

_____

_____

_____

November 25th

Thought of the Day

Kitchens that feed the homeless are over-run with volunteers at Thanksgiving time. My son and I have been some of those volunteers. We should continue to volunteer. However, we can't forget that people who need help need it all through the year and not just at the holidays. I think we get so much during the holiday season that we want to make sure those who are less fortunate get something as well. Consider spreading your generosity throughout the year. It will bless you and those with whom you spend your time.

My prayer for today is:

_____

_____

_____

What I am thankful for today:

_____

_____

_____

_____

My thoughts for today:

_____

_____

_____

_____

November 26th

Thought of the Day

I started cooking Thanksgiving meals for my family when my aunt and my grandmother began having health issues and couldn't keep up the tradition. They had been the cooks, and my mother would contribute dishes. I didn't know how good it would feel to keep the tradition going. The first time I called Grandmother to ask her how to cook something, she said to put in a "pinch" of this or that. It all turned out very well. I had absorbed more of their cooking prowess than I realized. It blessed me to be of help to them. Bring your contributions to the table whatever they are. Consider it a community table that blesses all who sit there.

My prayer for today is:

_____

_____

_____

What I am thankful for today:

_____

_____

_____

_____

My thoughts for today:

_____

_____

_____

_____

November 27th

Thought of the Day

When we're invited to someone else's home for Thanksgiving, do we bring something with us? The courteous thing is to do so. More importantly, do you bring a heart of thanksgiving? I think the best Thanksgiving Day dinners come with a generous side of gratitude.

My prayer for today is:

_____

_____

_____

What I am thankful for today:

_____

_____

_____

_____

My thoughts for today:

_____

_____

_____

_____

_____

November 28th

Thought of the Day

I always start Thanksgiving Day by watching the Macy's Thanksgiving Day Parade in New York City. Either the parade has been on my TV or I have actually been in New York to see it in person. The excitement is palpable as the big balloons are being inflated. Bands from all over the nation enter the city to represent their hometowns. Celebrities ride on the elaborate floats. A huge throng gathers along the streets to watch the parade. It's not about the ceremony of it. It's really about tradition. The best part of Thanksgiving tradition is the gathering of friends and family to share thanks over food made from recipes often passed down from one generation to the next. In that regard, Thanksgiving is really about "soul" food. I'm not speaking of a style of cooking but the fact that we are filled with love and gratitude for our fellowships. Be thankful today.

My prayer for today is:

_____

_____

_____

What I am thankful for today:

_____

_____

_____

_____

My thoughts for today:

_____

_____

_____

_____

November 29th

Thought of the Day

I can still remember a sermon from a guest minister from when I was a child. The minister preached for only 10 minutes or less, and the title of his sermon was Pass the SALT. S was for salvation. A is for the always-present God. L is because God lives. T is for being thankful for the gift of Jesus Christ. There will be lots of mentions of seasoning during this festive season filled with food. I pray that you have plenty of SALT.

My prayer for today is:

_____

_____

_____

What I am thankful for today:

_____

_____

_____

_____

My thoughts for today:

_____

_____

_____

_____

_____

November 30th

Thought of the Day

There is a song that so many people know. For others who may not have heard it, they quickly jump in. "Thank you, Lord. Thank you, Lord. Thank you, Lord. I just want to thank you, Lord." It's not unusual to see tears streaming down cheeks while it is being sung. It is simple but powerful. When there is nothing else you can say, when you are overwhelmed by gratitude, you can simply say, thank you, Lord.

My prayer for today is:

_____

_____

_____

What I am thankful for today:

_____

_____

_____

_____

My thoughts for today:

_____

_____

_____

_____

_____

December

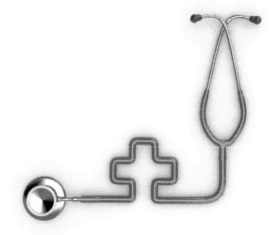

December
Christmas Gift

Medicine

In my opinion, December is a great month! I particularly love Christmas. The miracle of the birth of Jesus sends a powerful positive energy that fills the air. I love the decorated trees and traditions with family and friends rekindle wonderful memories. Many of my memories focus on my grandparents. They are all celebrating in heaven now. My maternal grandfather never met a stranger. He knew everyone. I imagine that he is still joking with my paternal grandfather who by comparison was not the greatest at remembering names.

I swear, my paternal grandmother was meant to be an orator. I'm pretty sure that she is not quiet even for a second in Heaven. Even though we would see my maternal grandmother on Christmas morning, we would call her first and she would say, "Christmas gift, Christmas gift. It's good to be alive. That's the Christmas gift!" We still greet each other within my family by calling on Christmas morning and repeating that sweet refrain.

It's not unusual to hear, "We wish you a Merry Christmas" as we're walking down grocery store aisles. I'm often singing along because I really do wish that for everyone I see. Unfortunately, Christmas is not merry for everyone. Some people experience seasonal depression. Feelings of sadness can come from stress associated with trying to finance a perfect holiday to feeling alone when everyone else seems to be celebrating togetherness. We seem to think we have to spread our joy at multiple households, exhausting ourselves into misery in the process. No matter the cause, that dreaded feeling is only compounded, as people feel more and more isolated in a cloud where they find no happiness. Those who feel this way may feel like they have to suffer in silence. Depression can convince you not to let anyone in, but it's masterfully deceptive in that it inhibits you from getting out. Reflect back over this entire year. The fact that you made it to the end of the year is a huge blessing. What have you accomplished this year? Focus on what was beautiful. Make the decision that not only will you end the year on a positive note but that you will take that spirit into the next year. The birth of Jesus is a Christmas gift that can break every chain. Allow yourself that gift. It's life-changing. What are you wanting for Christmas, preacher?

Ministry

I want everyone to think about the simplest blessings in life and then thank God for them. The holiday season is certainly my favorite time of year. However, with every birthday I celebrate, my perspective on what's truly important sharpens during the holidays. Certainly, for the kids, gifts galore and time out of school is premium. For me, the simplest things are the greatest things. Sure, I love gifts. But I'm a people person, so I love gatherings. I actually enjoy being out in the crowds. I often drive at night just to see decorations. However, I'm thankful that I can truly say that I'm at a point in life where the joy of Jesus means the most to me. Simply being with family and friends is a priceless gift. Down time from ministry and mediating on God and His goodness to me fills my heart. I "celebrate the simple" during the holidays now. Life. Health. A sound mind. True friendships. Making it through another year. The ability to laugh and love. All of these things and so much more truly bless me. I'm at a point where I can honestly say that if I don't get one material gift, being alive in Jesus satisfies me.

Conversely, I am fully aware that Christmas is not so festive for so many people for many reasons. I know that that the holidays can be stressful and downright depressing for many people. I know there is some grief, hurt, pain, and tears that come with the holidays for many. Believe me, I wish I could just say some "good church words" to make it all better. However, let me encourage those who suffer more than celebrate during the holidays to take a step back and think of small, simple things to be grateful for. For instance, no matter the trial, the Lord saw you through it. Think of the days early in the year or mid-year that making it to the end of the year mentally or emotionally seemed impossible. However, God kept you, held you, and helped you to make it. Most of all, think about how Jesus was born so He could die so that we all can live for God in the earth and live with God when life is over. These are reasons to celebrate. Celebrate true friends who were there for you. Celebrate small victories like going back to work or getting back into a great routine in church. Celebrate the fact that you can smile again and God's the one who restored it. Just know the same power that produced the miracle of the birth of Jesus is the same power that will birth a new day in your life.

My Year in Review

Our sincerest hope for you is that you will have peace and blessings beyond measure. Each month, we have asked you what your goals are. This month, we're asking you to reflect on what you've achieved this year.

1.

2.

3.

December 1st

Thought of the Day

Have you watched the movie, *It's a Wonderful Life*. It's a classic at Christmas time. The main character laments his existence until he gets to witness what life would be like without him. He comes to realize that there is value in his life not only for himself but for others he positively impacted. His troubles clouded his being able to see how it was not a mistake that he was meant to be on this earth for many reasons. Likewise, there is too much value in your life for you not to believe in yourself.

My prayer for today is:

_____

_____

_____

What is the gift I'm thankful for today:

_____

_____

_____

_____

My thoughts for today:

_____

_____

_____

_____

_____

December 2nd

Thought of the Day

Sometimes God uses the difficulties in our lives as a heavenly steering wheel to keep us turning and coming right back to Him over and over again. So don't worry about the temporary noise and shaking that life's potholes may present to you. It's all worth it to arrive safely at the feet of the One who has passion and power to do exactly what you need Him to do.

My prayer for today is:

_____

_____

_____

What is the gift I'm thankful for today:

_____

_____

_____

_____

My thoughts for today:

_____

_____

_____

_____

_____

December 3rd

Thought of the Day

I just saw a story on the news about a puppy named Rudolph in Oklahoma that was administered euthanasia because the rescue shelter he was in was overcrowded. Miraculously, Rudolph WOKE UP after a few minutes! Rudolph refused to die! There will be times when some might discount you as useless and not worth it. There will always be situations that seem to take the breath and life out of you. But pull a Rudolph! Refuse to die! His story ends by a man coming and adopting him to take care of him forever. Well, through Jesus, we've been adopted, too! We have a Father in heaven who loves us and will keep us forever!

My prayer for today is:

_____

_____

_____

What is the gift I'm thankful for today:

_____

_____

_____

_____

My thoughts for today:

_____

_____

_____

_____

_____

December 4th

Thought of the Day

We must learn and grow in God to the point where we totally trust Him. When we arrive at that spiritual place, we'll genuinely, wholeheartedly praise Him for what HE'S GOING TO DO before He ever does it. When we truly trust and believe, we'll thank Him in advance for His blessings, deliverance, provision, and assistance.

My prayer for today is:

_____

_____

_____

What is the gift I'm thankful for today:

_____

_____

_____

_____

My thoughts for today:

_____

_____

_____

_____

_____

December 5ᵗʰ

Thought of the Day

The Christmas gift that I used to love giving more than any other was the one I used to give to Buck. Buck was a gentle-spirited man who was too often discounted because he struggled with illiteracy. He took care of his aunt until her passing. His mode of transportation was his bike. He was dependable and kind. He used to bring us kids candy on days he would ride into town. At Christmas, he didn't have much to give but he would buy tokens anyway. It did my heart good to give him presents because he appreciated them so much. I gave him everything from cologne to a Walmart gift card that he could use to get things he needed. He told people he could go into Walmart and get anything he wanted for life because I had given him a card. He had misunderstood. I hadn't given him a $1 million gift card, but it flattered me that he knew I would make sure he had what he needed. Truth be told, I would have filled that card over and over again because I did want to make sure he was taken care of. He passed away so I didn't have that opportunity. It still warms my heart to think of Buck. He gave me more than I gave him. Encounters with genuine people are better gifts than expensive gifts from fake people.

My prayer for today is:

_____

_____

_____

What is the gift I'm thankful for today:

_____

_____

_____

_____

My thoughts for today:

_____

_____

_____

_____

_____

December 6th

Thought of the Day

Bil Keane, American cartoonist of *The Family Circle*, said, "Yesterday is history, tomorrow is a mystery, today is a gift of God, which is why we call it the present." Open your present today and do something great with it!

My prayer for today is:

_____

_____

_____

What is the gift I'm thankful for today:

_____

_____

_____

My thoughts for today:

_____

_____

_____

_____

December 7th

Thought of the Day

I was watching Major League Baseball highlights one night when something came to mind. The pitcher never throws his pitch until the catcher faces him, squats, and holds his mitt up, signaling that he's ready to receive the pitch. Could it be that God is delaying His release of some blessings designed for us because we're not in position and ready to receive them? Assume your upright position by praying, studying His Word, obeying His directions, praising Him, worshipping Him, and walking in faith. Then watch God release what heaven has in store for you.

My prayer for today is:

_____

_____

_____

What is the gift I'm thankful for today:

_____

_____

_____

_____

My thoughts for today:

_____

_____

_____

_____

_____

December 8th

Thought of the Day

Never be ashamed of what God is doing in your life. There is a difference between celebrating God and being conceited. Being grateful looks a lot different than thinking you are the one who is great. Let others label you and your successes as they wish. But you never lose sight of the fact that if God hadn't done it, it wouldn't have been done. You're about praise and not pretense! Don't pay attention to those who don't know the difference. Walk in your blessings.

My prayer for today is:

_____

_____

_____

What is the gift I'm thankful for today:

_____

_____

_____

My thoughts for today:

_____

_____

_____

_____

December 9th

Thought of the Day

Faith 101. Faith is celebrating your complete healing while still hurting and waiting to hear the final report and plan from the doctor. Faith believes the blessing is coming long before your eyes can behold the blessing. Faith is believing you'll lose enough weight to come off your medications. Faith is sticking with the treatment to relieve your depression. Faith is knowing God will deliver through whatever channel He ordains. It's not about asking how. Faith is about believing and being open to receiving. Believe and receive!

My prayer for today is:

_____

_____

_____

What is the gift I'm thankful for today:

_____

_____

_____

My thoughts for today:

_____

_____

_____

_____

December 10th

Thought of the Day

True peace is arriving at the point spiritually and mentally where it really doesn't matter what or who you face because you know that God has the ultimate say in everything concerning you. This peace allows you to truly view every obstacle as just another opportunity for God to be God in your life. Let God work on your behalf. Wishing you peace and joy!

My prayer for today is:

_____

_____

_____

What is the gift I'm thankful for today:

_____

_____

_____

_____

My thoughts for today:

_____

_____

_____

_____

December 11th

Thought of the Day

Complaining is a great stall tactic of Satan. He uses our complaints to stall our concentration on where we are rather than looking at where we're going. He also uses complaints to stall our ambitions at "what happened" rather than allowing us to believe what God will make happen in our lives and for our lives. Keep your complaints. Keep your composure. Then keep living life until dreams are realized, goals are achieved, and hindrances are overcome.

My prayer for today is:

_____

_____

_____

What is the gift I'm thankful for today:

_____

_____

_____

_____

My thoughts for today:

_____

_____

_____

_____

December 12th

Thought of the Day

Sometimes your healing can come by way of helping others. People don't always need you to "do" something. They may just need you to be near them and for you to be you. If they can see God in how you move at that moment, they are comforted. The simple gift of presence is sometimes the best present you can give anyone.

My prayer for today is:

_____

_____

_____

What is the gift I'm thankful for today:

_____

_____

_____

_____

My thoughts for today:

_____

_____

_____

_____

_____

December 13th

Thought of the Day

The holidays are one of those times we don't like to look at the dreaded scale. Look at it now so you're not surprised at the beginning of the new year. Enjoy the cheer. You can eat and drink—in moderation. Practice the exercise of smiling and laughing this holiday season. Turn off the phone and the TV at night so you can get some sleep. Don't overspend on gifts. The gift people want most of all is to have you around for many years to come.

My prayer for today is:

_____

_____

_____

What is the gift I'm thankful for today:

_____

_____

_____

_____

My thoughts for today:

_____

_____

_____

_____

_____

December 14th

Thought of the Day

Friend, no matter how it feels, looks, or seems, the truth is that a praise break is always warranted. It may not seem like it at the moment, but things could be worse than what they are now. So thank God for sustaining you and covering you no matter what's affecting you right now. Celebrate that things are as well as they are and believe by faith that things will be better.

My prayer for today is:

_____

_____

_____

What is the gift I'm thankful for today:

_____

_____

_____

_____

My thoughts for today:

_____

_____

_____

_____

_____

December 15th

Thought of the Day

To depend on God is to defer all of your concerns, issues, and problems to Him, knowing there is nothing that He can't or won't handle. When you give Him your concerns, go on about your business, glorifying Him for who He is and for what He's about to do. His gift is on the way!

My prayer for today is:

_____

_____

_____

What is the gift I'm thankful for today:

_____

_____

_____

_____

My thoughts for today:

_____

_____

_____

_____

_____

December 16th

Thought of the Day

God is greater and stronger than your greatest and strongest challenge, dilemma, enemy, or situation. When you know this and believe this, you have a battle cry that keeps you going: I'VE GOT THE VICTORY! Turn whatever or whomever concerns you over to God today.

My prayer for today is:

_____

_____

_____

What is the gift I'm thankful for today:

_____

_____

_____

My thoughts for today:

_____

_____

_____

_____

December 17th

Thought of the Day

This morning, I discovered that I neglected to activate our home security system before going to bed last night. I have protection; yet I failed to apply it. That's just about as useless as having God's Word, hearing God's Word, shouting about God's Word, teaching and preaching God's Word, reciting God's Word, and then neglecting to apply it to our lives. God's Word and God's Spirit are available to lead us, guide us, inspire us, convict us, and change us. However, without application, we are uncovered, unprotected, often unsettled, and unstable. Cover yourself safely in the blanket of God's love.

My prayer for today is:

_____

_____

_____

What is the gift I'm thankful for today:

_____

_____

_____

_____

My thoughts for today:

_____

_____

_____

_____

_____

December 18th

Thought of the Day

Even though we try to figure God out, our minds are not capable of comprehending the goodness or the greatness of God nor the depth of His grace toward us. We serve an incredible God who deserves incredible praise and worship from us! A wonderful day is all yours, knowing that you are a recipient of His gift of grace.

My prayer for today is:

_____

_____

_____

What is the gift I'm thankful for today:

_____

_____

_____

My thoughts for today:

_____

_____

_____

_____

December 19th

Thought of the Day

You will never be able to control "them." Just be concerned with taking full control of yourself. Whatever you do, don't give others control over you! Don't let anyone steal your joy in this season. After all, that seat of authority, power, and control should be given to God and God only! Surrender to your Savior and not to your surroundings!

My prayer for today is:

_____

_____

_____

What is the gift I'm thankful for today:

_____

_____

_____

_____

My thoughts for today:

_____

_____

_____

_____

_____

December 20th

Thought of the Day

God will certainly be a "fence" around us each day. However, it's not His fault if we unlatch the gate and walk out of the safety of His fence. The blessings of the Lord hinge more on our discipline than they do on God doing something. I don't know about you, I just want to be wherever the Lord is. Thank God for peace and safety.

My prayer for today is:

_____

_____

_____

What is the gift I'm thankful for today:

_____

_____

_____

_____

My thoughts for today:

_____

_____

_____

_____

_____

December 21st

Thought of the Day

The best blessing of this day is that you lived to see it. Sometimes we are searching for big miracles and we ignore the miracles that happen every day. This wouldn't be a wellness journal if I didn't point out that you have the wonderful, amazing opportunity to incorporate some wellness into your day so you can see many more sunrises. Each day is a gift and an opportunity. Now live each moment to its fullest.

My prayer for today is:

_____

_____

_____

What is the gift I'm thankful for today:

_____

_____

_____

My thoughts for today:

_____

_____

_____

_____

December 22nd

Thought of the Day

I have lights strung up on my house yearly for the Christmas season. I have an arrangement whereby a company stores my lights, comes out regularly each year in late November, and puts the lights up that trim my house. I go to work and come home one day and the lights are up. They are beautiful. But even their light can't outshine my smile when I see them. I think they make me so happy because I'm showing everyone around me that I unashamedly celebrate the season. It often spurs conversations where I can share that I love Christmas not only for the decorations themselves but for how the decorations are tied to the true meaning of the season for my life. It's so funny now because I will have neighbors text me at work to say, "Guess what? Your lights are going up." Let your celebration of the birth of Jesus be contagious!

My prayer for today is:

_____

_____

_____

What is the gift I'm thankful for today:

_____

_____

_____

_____

My thoughts for today:

_____

_____

_____

_____

December 23rd

Thought of the Day

I watch *Merry Christmas Charlie Brown* every year! You might guess that if you saw the little Charlie Brown tree I have as part of my décor. Thank goodness, Linus reminds the Peanuts gang of the true meaning of Christmas. He schooled them and then they wrap their love around what was a pitiful-looking tree turning it into a magnificent tree. That preaches to me every time! Let the true meaning of love not only fill you up but overflow in you so that you bless somebody else.

My prayer for today is:

_____

_____

_____

What is the gift I'm thankful for today:

_____

_____

_____

_____

My thoughts for today:

_____

_____

_____

_____

_____

December 24th

Thought of the Day

I love Christmas eve! Most of the stores close early so that the temptation for more shopping ceases. I tend to bake a few goodies for the next day. My favorite part is watching the lights dance on the tree. The shining star on my tree reminds me of the star that guided the wise men to the baby Jesus. The tranquility from resetting myself to focus on the true meaning of the season makes me smile as I listen to the Temptations sing *Silent Night*. May glories stream on you from heaven afar!

My prayer for today is:

_____

_____

_____

What is the gift I'm thankful for today:

_____

_____

_____

_____

My thoughts for today:

_____

_____

_____

_____

December 25th

Thought of the Day

Christmas gift! Christmas gift! I love the joy that comes from watching children open their gifts. Their exuberance is priceless. I doubt they see the joy we have in watching them. I know they don't see how grateful we are that our biggest presents come from knowing that we are blessed enough to have everything we need and even a little more to get them some of the things they want. Even though they don't see it, let's make sure we let God know that we are thankful for His Christmas gifts.

My prayer for today is:

_____

_____

_____

What is the gift I'm thankful for today:

_____

_____

_____

My thoughts for today:

_____

_____

_____

_____

December 26th

Thought of the Day

When God is truly your EVERYTHING, then you don't have to worry about ANYTHING because He can and will handle all things for you. Keep your faith focus. Walk confidently knowing that His promises are yea and amen! What wonderful gifts!

My prayer for today is:

_____

_____

_____

What is the gift I'm thankful for today:

_____

_____

_____

_____

My thoughts for today:

_____

_____

_____

_____

_____

December 27th

Thought of the Day

Once Christmas is over, some of us feel depleted. It's like there was so much build-up to this one day, and then it's over. We are already yearning for something else to look forward to. Others of us are glad it's over because it was viewed as stressful. The real gift of Christmas should make us glad and last for the entire year. Don't let the trappings of the holiday season trap you in emotions. Focus on the Word of God, which will liberate you to celebrate at all times.

My prayer for today is:

_____

_____

_____

What is the gift I'm thankful for today:

_____

_____

_____

My thoughts for today:

_____

_____

_____

_____

December 28th

Thought of the Day

I hate returning a gift that someone gave me for Christmas. It's not only because I hate the absolute chaos in the stores after Christmas, but it's because I value the sentiment behind the gift. I do have to realize that if the gift is totally wrong for me or doesn't work, it won't serve any good purpose. I won't be able to use it, and the giver will have wasted money for something that I'll have to put in a closet. So, I will make that return and make sure the giver knows I am able to put their generosity to use. As we prepare to go into the new year, there may be some things you have to leave behind to move purposefully ahead in the new year. It's okay because the wisdom and knowledge from lessons learned are gifts that keep giving.

My prayer for today is:

_____

_____

_____

What is the gift I'm thankful for today:

_____

_____

_____

_____

My thoughts for today:

_____

_____

_____

_____

_____

December 29th

Thought of the Day

I gave my family—adults and children alike—nuts, apples, oranges, and peppermints in commemorative cups last year for Christmas. The cups said, "Christmas Gift." That gift brought up memories of the fruit bowls on Grandmother's table that had been a part of our Christmas tradition growing up. Sometimes it's the small gestures that mean so much. The small gestures are often symbols of great love. There were times in my grandparents' lives when they didn't have much to give, so it really was the thought that counted. I am thankful that our grandparents planted seeds of faith and gratitude in us. We'll keep passing that gift on.

My prayer for today is:

_____

_____

_____

What is the gift I'm thankful for today:

_____

_____

_____

_____

My thoughts for today:

_____

_____

_____

_____

December 30th

Thought of the Day

Sometimes when we go to football games, we leave at the end of the third quarter. We think we've seen enough to know what will happen. We hurry to our car and turn on the radio to listen to the remainder of the game while driving home. Imagine our surprise when the game takes a turn that we weren't expecting! It's the same with life. Sometimes we think we know the outcome because of what we've seen. Even though we're coming to the end of the year, hold on to your faith because it is not too late for God to turn things around on your behalf. Don't count yourself out! I believe that God can still present you with a win.

My prayer for today is:

_____

_____

_____

What is the gift I'm thankful for today:

_____

_____

_____

_____

My thoughts for today:

_____

_____

_____

_____

_____

December 31st

Thought of the Day

We've made it to the end of a year. We see many recaps of the year, including the best songs of the year, the most popular news headlines, and even people we lost that year. There are always highs and lows. What does your recap look like? Did your good days outweigh your bad days? It's cool to recount the milestones of this past year but also let them be the stepping stones to even better days ahead in the upcoming year. Be blessed!

My prayer for today is:

_____

_____

_____

What is the gift I'm thankful for today:

_____

_____

_____

_____

My thoughts for today:

_____

_____

_____

_____

_____

Epilogue

Medicine

Throughout this journal, we hope that we have encouraged you on your journey. Prayerfully, you have found additional strength for your journey. That strength didn't come from our words but from what's already inside of you. Even if you have had to stumble along the way, get up and keep going! It was intentional that different perspectives were presented because different perspectives matter. No one approach works for everyone, and everyone needs to be heard. We hope that we have started a conversation that you will continue. We could have called this *When Ministry Clashes with Medicine*. However, we felt like it was more appropriately titled *When Ministry Meets Medicine* because the goal of both is healing. Isn't that right, preacher?

Ministry

You're absolutely correct. The truth is, when we began this project, I felt that there would be more clashes than meetings. However, if you've read this journal thoroughly, you've found more meetings than clashes. That's because, as the good doctor stated, our goal is to provide dialogue that will lead you to a place of healing, wholeness, and restoration.

My sister is a doggone good medical professional. As of this writing, I'm a preacher of 22 years and a pastor of 19 years. The good doctor's life centers a ton on medical facts. My life centers mostly on the Master's scriptures. When discussing situations—often like Matthew, Mark, Luke, and John—we speak from our particular prisms of expertise. However, she's not void of faith.

I'm not ignorant or dismissive of facts. The beauty of all this hinges in one centrally focused place: Jesus. We both love Jesus. We both believe God has the final say in all things. We also both believe that we, as believers, have a say in what happens to us and for us as well. After reading these entries, our hope is that you agree with us!

About the Authors

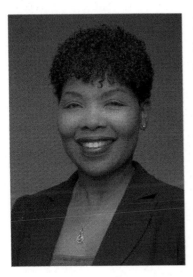

Dr. Andrea Green Willis was born in Athens, Alabama where her family continues to reside. She graduated from Athens High School and completed her undergraduate work at the University of Alabama at Birmingham. She continued her education by pursuing a medical degree from Georgetown University School of Medicine. She also obtained her Master of Public Health from Johns Hopkins. Dr. Willis is currently a board-certified pediatrician.

She was recognized by Modern Healthcare as one of 2018's Top 25 Minority Executives in Healthcare and one of the 50 Most Influential Clinical Executives in 2019. Johns Hopkins recognized her as a distinguished alumna in 2019.

Dr. Willis is a dedicated member at Mount Zion Baptist Church in Nashville, Tennessee, and she is a proud mother of one son, Cameron, who is currently attending New York University.

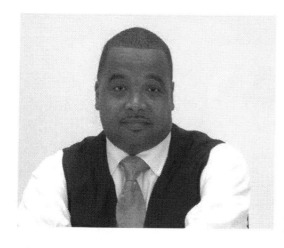

Antoyne L. Green is the Senior Pastor of New Life Church in Athens, Alabama. He has served in this capacity since June 2000 as a proud Athens-Limestone native.

Pastor Green attained a Bachelor of Arts degree in broadcast journalism with a minor in history at the University of Alabama in Tuscaloosa. Upon graduating, he worked as a news anchor and reporter at WCFT and WDBB television stations in Tuscaloosa. He also worked at WBRC Fox 6 News in Birmingham until he assumed the pastorate full time.

Pastor Green currently spends much of his time teaching and preaching the gospel in various venues across the country. He's also an accomplished author with three books to his credit: *A Closer Walk With God: One Day at a Time*, *However Tte Lord Chooses: He May Not Do it Your Way*, and *Decisions: My Head vs. My Heart*.

Pastor Green is married to the former Felicia Batts of Huntsville. They have three children: Jasmynn, Kaleb, and Emani.

Stay in Touch

Our Website: www.whenministrymeetsmedicine.com
Book us to Speak: www.whenministrymeetsmedicine.com/booking
You can find us on Instagram @whenministrymeetsmedicine and Twitter @minmeetsmed

Made in the USA
Lexington, KY
05 December 2019

58188000R00249